DECISIONS AND DILEMMAS IN CARE HOMES

DECISIONS AND DILEMMAS IN CARE HOMES

Carol Dimon
RN, DIPN, BSc (Hons) Nursing studies, MMEDSCI, PGCE

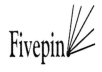

Fivepin Limited, 92 Crane Street, Salisbury, Wiltshire, SP1 2PU
www.fivepin.co.uk

British Library Cataloguing in Publication Data
A catalogue record for this book is available from the British Library

©Fivepin 2006
ISBN: 1 9038 7743 1

Printed in the UK by Lightning Source, Milton Keynes

Dedication

In memory of my sister Helen McSweeney.

For my children Rachel and Joshua so they may live in a more caring society.

Acknowledgements

With thanks to Lynette Chipp, my typist and editor, who worked so hard.

Elsie, aged 92, is in tears. Why?

A nurse has just removed a chocolate éclair from her hand because Elsie is on a reducing diet.

This book is written for Elsie and residents like her, who are in a state of distress.

It is also written for nurses and care assistants to encourage thinking.

CONTENTS

Foreword

If any of us ever have to move into a care home we will be faced with one of life's major transitions.

Moving may entail the loss of home, social contacts, and pets. We may have to discard treasured possessions because of lack of space. We might have to enter residential care following an illness or other major trauma that has resulted in a decline in our physical or mental abilities. In other words, the transition to residential care might involve the loss of all the things that we rely on for a sense of safety and security. Our move might be made straight from hospital and at very short notice. Once in a home we are likely to find ourselves in an almost uniquely powerless position. We will have no security of tenure, if we are in an independent sector home we will be not protected by the Human Rights Act, and if we have no relatives or friends who visit us we may have little contact with the outside world.

Working in a care home is therefore about much more than meeting the physical needs of residents for care and attention. Staff need to work in a way that restores the dignity and sense of worth and security that the transition to long term care may have stripped away.

The new White Paper on Health and Social Care, *Our Health, Our Care, Our Say*, presents all staff working in care homes with a major challenge as it seeks to draw health and social care values together in order to address the needs of the 'whole person'. 'We will bring skill development frameworks together and create career pathways across health and social care', says the White Paper.

Staff will be helped to 'develop skills that are portable, based on shared values, recognised across the sectors and built around the needs of patients and service users', These proposals have the potential to lead to a more highly trained social care workforce, but they also have the potential to revolutionise the culture and values of health based professions such as nursing, with the focus moving towards 'supporting people through their life journey', as Beverly Malone put it at a launch event for the White Paper.

Decisions and Dilemmas in Care Homes is based on the premise that staff who work in residential homes are constantly required to make decisions that involve respect for the dignity and rights of a fellow citizen. Everyday decisions – such as how to respond to a resident who does not want to go on an outing, or a resident who wants to bath alone - and internal policies, such as restrictions on smoking or use of alcohol – all require consideration of the resident as a whole person, and recognition of the extent to which decisions can undermine both the autonomy and dignity of the resident. Age Concern commends this approach as contributing to just the type of change in the values of social care and nursing that the White Paper promises.

Gordon Lishman

1   INTRODUCTION

A vast range of skills is required to deliver care within care homes. This area of care sadly lacks public and professional recognition (Reed and Stanley, 2003) and is often criticised for low standards of care. This book aims to illustrate the skills that are required within care homes by exploring the many challenges that confront nurses and care assistants.

Based upon experiences within long-term care establishments as a registered nurse, the author has identified various dilemmas of care. These shall be referred to as issues defined as controversial situations that may create conflicts between nurses, care assistants or other professionals, nurses and residents or relatives. There are no legal or professional guidelines referring specifically to them and they may arise spontaneously. Such issues are not confined to long-term care or to specific areas of care and they may arise within the most innovative areas. However, they may be more evident within long-term care because residents and staff may be present for a greater length of time and the residents are more likely to be of a vulnerable nature. Whatever action is taken, a reason is always provided by the nurse or care assistant when questioned. Different staff, however, may provide different rationales which the resident may not always be aware of or in agreement with. Hence the author will consider issues individually, outlining possible actions that may or may not be taken. This book does not aim to prescribe action. It will, however, be a useful reference tool or teaching aid, serving as a guide to nurses, stimulating thinking and standard setting. This book is written primarily for all staff within nursing or residential homes who are constantly confronted by decisions.

There are various issues, some of which may prevail historically. This book refers to the daily decisions arising within care homes:

1

Introduction

- Daily decisions refer to those decisions concerning daily aspects of care, for example washing or dressing.
- Clinical decisions refer to such as wound care.
- Managerial decisions refer to issues concerning management of care and the home, such as disciplining staff.

Whilst reference is made to nurses only throughout the book, it also applies to care assistants and senior care assistants.

2 BACKGROUND

Care homes are essential within our society, providing care for residents including older people, and people with mental illnesses, with physical disabilities or with learning difficulties. They may be owned by private companies or individuals, charities or the NHS.

Figures for care homes are very difficult to obtain. There are 29,890 care homes in the UK (Laing and Buisson, 2005). Despite present government policy to increase care in the community (Dinsdale and Parish, 2005) there will always be a need for care homes. However, the dependency of residents in care homes is consequently increasing.

Whilst nursing and residential homes are now collectively referred to as care homes according to the Care Standards Act 2000, there is a difference between them. Nursing homes theoretically care for more dependant residents and a nurse must be on duty every shift. In England, the Care Standards Act requires the registered manager to be nurse.

Residential homes are not required to be managed by a nurse. Senior care assistants may manage them. All managers must have at least two years experience in a senior management capacity in a relevant care setting (Care Standards Act 2000). Prior to this Act, no previous experience or training was legally required.

If a resident in a residential home requires nursing care, this is provided by the district nurse. In some cases, the district nurse may train the senior care assistant to perform dressings or insulin injections for example. There is thus a distinction between social care such as bathing, and nursing care such as doing dressings. Before admission, all individuals are assessed according to this (Department of Health 2005). However, there may be misplacement of residents into either nursing or residential care. For example, a resident in a

3

residential home may really need nursing care (Nazarko, 1999).

Figures for staff in care homes are unavailable. However, some figures are available for the general social care workforce (Skills for Care 2005). It is stated that there are over 70,000 nurses working in nursing homes (Nazarko 1995).

Care assistants are the majority of the workforce. Therefore, they are in a position to make decisions. As yet they are not registered as professionals, in the same way as nurses, (Department of Health 2004) other than under the Protection of Vulnerable Adults Register. A code of practice does exist for care assistants (General Social Care Workforce 2002) addressing such aspects as training and policies.

Training needs for all care staff have been addressed by the Care Standards (2003). At least 50 per cent of all care assistants must possess NVQ 2 or 3 by 2005. Managers of care homes must have at least NVQ 4 in management or the equivalent by 2005. All staff must undertake the equivalent of three days training a year. Indeed, there is mandatory training such as fire, and health and safety.

The need for a nurse at all in care homes has been debated for a number of years (Dimon, 1995). Indeed there is a national shortage of nurses. Many homes employ foreign nurses, having assisted them with their adaptation (O'Dowd, 2003).

Homes are inspected by members of the Commission for Social Care Inspection team in England and Wales according to the Care Standards (2003). Whilst these standards do address such issues as choice, they are interpreted in different ways by different inspectors (English Community Care Association, 2004), for example in the evaluation of care plans. There is little research available as yet regarding this. The Commission for Social Care Inspection will be joining the Health Care Commission in 2008 (Age Concern Bulletin, 2005).

In Scotland, homes are inspected by the Scottish Commission for the Regulation of Scottish Care Standards (Cooper, 2003). In Northern Ireland, homes are inspected by the Registration and Inspection Unit and standards are presently being developed.

Decisions and Dilemmas in Care Homes

It must be remembered that the registered manager has ultimate responsibility for the care within the home, even though the registered nurse is accountable for his or her own actions (NMC, 2004). This means that if a nurse or care assistant makes the wrong decision, the home manager will be involved in an investigation. Therefore it is important that the home manager is aware of decisions that are being made, particularly as documented within the care plan.

The development of care homes is not helped by the difficulty in obtaining background information. It would be beneficial if the information was collated by some agency. This may be enabled by the progression of the Commission for Social Care Inspection.

3   REGULATIONS

There are various regulations which influence care in care homes.

Human Rights Act (1998)

This allows individuals to dispute issues in UK courts, instead of the European Court in Strasbourg. Rights in this Act which may have particular relevance to care homes include:

- Right to liberty and security;
- Right to respect for private and family life;
- Freedom of thought, conscience and religion.

Indeed a number of care home cases involving this Act have reached the courts, for example a case regarding a resident who had to be moved to another care home due to her increased needs (Age Concern Bulletin, October 2004).

Care Standards Act (2000).

This Act replaced the Registered Homes Act (1984) for England and Wales. It announced national standards. The standards refer to such topics as medication, care plans, autonomy and choice.

Code of Practice – General Social Care Council 2002

This code, for social care workers and their employers, describes required standards. Statements refer to rights, trust, independence and safety of residents.

The NMC Code of Conduct 2002

This code is the professional code for registered nurses and it governs the standard of their practice. Points such as 'respect the patient as an individual' and 'minimise the risk to patients' are highly relevant to this book.

Health and Safety Act 1974

This Act and subsequent regulations govern health and safety of equipment, buildings and individuals. It highlights the importance of undertaking individual assessments. It addresses fire and manual handling and specifies legal requirements; all of these have relevance to this book.

4 HISTORICAL ISSUES

Historical exploration of caring in care homes will indicate any possible foundation for the decisions and dilemmas that arise.

Elderly people were a majority of the workhouse population (Rose, 1971; Crowther, 1981; Longmate, 1974) being classified as poor amongst criminals, children, insane and unmarried mothers according to the Poor Law Act 1601 and its amendments 1834. Whilst this is disputed (Thompson, 1983) based upon available records, similar issues arose within workhouses to nursing homes possibly because they both involve the provision of residence. Therefore the examination of historical issues shall commence with reference to the workhouses.

Within the workhouse era, care was a deterrent against state dependency because poverty was considered to be self-induced but conditions did vary and were worse within parish areas which were smaller and less wealthy (Rose, 1971). A uniform regime was maintained regarding meal or bedtimes; games or books were not permitted, razors were not permitted, baths were weekly in the presence of staff and inmates had to apply for permission to go out (Crowther, 1981). There was an absence of furniture or cutlery and workhouses were overcrowded, with inmates sharing a bed. It was argued that they would share a bed at home anyway (Crowther, 1981). Males and females were separated, mother and child were separated in some cases and husband and wife were punished if they spoke. This was to prevent habitation, expansion of the poverty race and influence of children and it was argued some preferred living apart (Longmate, 1974). Punishments were issued for being noisy or dirty, swearing or refusing to work and included restriction of food, increased workload or solitary confinement (Crowther, 1981). Medical consent was, however, required to punish the elderly or pregnant. Work consisted of weaving or grinding, for example. Visitors were not permitted until the 1850s when L. Twining established a voluntary visiting committee (Crowther, 1981). This was later replaced by the House committees in 1913 which were to spend small amounts of money without guardians' consent. Visits were then permitted for one hour during the afternoon. Guardians possessed the major authority above workhouse masters, appointing staff and managing finances, and therefore the government was unable to enforce alterations (Smith, 1977). However, guardians were mainly businessmen or farmers and possessed little knowledge of institutions. Master and matron who was not a nurse were usually married and therefore in close alliance.

Inspections were undertaken by Poor Law commissioners but were infrequent and inadequate. Unannounced visits and an advisory approach were suggested but not adopted (Rose, 1971). From 1913 records of complaints were kept but dismissed staff were able to obtain work within other locations. The workhouses were renamed Poor Law institutions signifying a change in approach. It was considered that pampering the elderly may influence the care of paupers. Such an approach was influenced by social conditions at the time; for example, floggings and executions were still common until 1865 (Lane, 1993). Attempts were made to humanise treatment, for example one workhouse master provided the elderly with separate teapots in 1860 but they were broken by inspectors because they were not in keeping with a deterrent approach (Longmate, 1974).

There were exceptions; for example, J. Carey in the 1860s in Bristol regarded care as shelter not a deterrent and provided a better diet (Longmate, 1974). Tuke during the 1800s provided more humanistic care, for example reduced restraint within a mental asylum based upon the religious Quaker philosophy of brotherhood.

The majority of staff were uneducated due to lack of recognition of an educational need, low salaries and unattractive work. The need for education was recognised during the 1850s encouraged by F. Nightingale. However, guardians restricted the employment of paid nurses, considering their duties to be those of inmates (Crowther,

1981). In 1870s probationers were employed with one year's instruction from medical officers and the head nurse, although the only requirement was for nurses to be able to read instructions, to be sober, motherly and kind.

A number of factors contributed towards improvement. There was increasing concern for the chronic sick within workhouses particularly concerning the death of a pauper (Crowther, 1981). Medical officers' ability to complain was strengthened by the establishment of, the Poor Law Medical Officers Association, founded 1868, British Medical Association 1832, the Lancet Journal and The Hospital Journals began in 1886 (Crowther, 1981). This promoted the establishment of the Association for Workhouse Improvements of Poor Law Infirmaries in 1866. The Association for Promoting Trained Nursing in Workhouse Infirmaries was established in 1879 (Crowther, 1981) but this soon ended because work within workhouses was unattractive due to low salaries, poor facilities and the chronic cases that they were getting due to voluntary hospitals' refusal to take them.

There has historically been a debate regarding the separation of specific groups of residents, for example children, mentally ill and elderly. In 1867 separate provision for the sick and insane was established which became county hospitals in 1930. However, separations were halted by the First World War (Crowther, 1981) during which inmates were distributed to other parishes and the number of inspections reduced. Two reports of Booth and Rowntree indicated that poverty was not self-induced but caused by unemployment, low wages and old age (Rose, 1971). As a result, the Royal Commission for aged poor was established in 1895 following which privileges were provided for the elderly including their own tea making ingredients, and lockers but staff kept the keys, tobacco on medical grounds, mixed gender day rooms, outings out alone and individual bed or mealtimes (Longmate, 1974). Two conflicting reports recommended the closure or improvement of workhouses (Royal Commission in Rose, 1971) but no action was taken. In 1908 the Old Age Pension Act was commenced but pensions were insufficient to prevent all of the elderly from requiring workhouses.

Professional developments of nursing also influenced

workhouses, for example State Registered Nurse (SRN) 1919, General Nursing Council (GNC) 1929, Royal College of Nursing (RCN) 1916 (Smith, 1977). However, the earlier probationary role indicated acknowledgement of different educational requirements. There had been a suggestion to combine care within workhouses with district nursing (Crowther, 1981). The image of the workhouses as a deterrent was reinforced by the general strike in 1916 lasting one week and the miners strike lasting for six months. Indeed some unions became bankrupt in 1928 resulting in the abolition of guardians, and allocation of authority to the councils. Workhouse inmates were transferred to their own home or other unions during the Second World War (Means and Smith, 1983) and many gathered within air raid shelters. Hence evacuation hostels were established particularly by the religious Quaker association. Following the war establishments were regarded as hotels and inmates as residents (Means and Smith, 1983) because the elderly were regarded as being innocently homeless. However, they were unlike hotels in any other way, for example in the degree of privacy permitted, but residents were provided with their own money, paying social services for their care. Workhouses were dissolved by the NHS Act 1946 and the National Assistance Act 1948, promoting the use of hospitals and residential homes. Common issues within workhouses referred to:

- Bathing;
- Bed or Mealtimes;
- Possession of games or books;
- Possession of own razors;
- Punishments;
- Privileges;
- Separation of male and female;
- Tobacco;
- Overcrowding;
- Visitors.

Whilst workhouse buildings existed ten years after the National Assistance Act, they were used as chronic hospitals or local authority homes, and no central records were kept.

Issues as identified by Townsend (1964) will be outlined because he was the major analyst at the time and his work referred to both nursing and residential homes. There were variations between types of home which were voluntarily, privately or publicly owned. Voluntary homes, including charity or religious homes, were considered to be more liberal for example permitting residents to bath alone (Townsend, 1964). Similar issues to workhouses remained evident despite such variations. Very few homes permitted the use of residents' own furniture due to lack of storage space. Use of residents' own clothes was discouraged, due to staff inconvenience for example. Good behaviour was rewarded by cigarettes for example and homes possessed a list of rules such as refraining from using obscene language. Baths were usually supervised by staff but no reason is provided for this. Residents were not permitted to make or serve their own drinks. Pocket money was limited if given because residents were said to be unable to deal with it. Residents were discouraged from assisting each other but no reason is provided for this.

Similar issues are outlined regarding care of the mentally ill (Goffman 1961) and reinforced by more recent reports (Meacher, 1972; Clough, 1981; Wade *et al*, 1983). Additional rationales are provided, for example residents own furniture would create a fire risk and risk of woodworm as well as lack of storage space (Willcocks *et al*, 1987). Residents were discouraged from using their own wardrobe to prevent excess laundry and untidiness (Meacher, 1972). There are also additional issues, for example possession of their own door keys was not permitted (Booth, 1985; Counsel and Care, 1992) and toilet doors were not lockable or locked (Clough, 1981). Residents were discouraged from making their own bed to prevent the introduction of fleas and to ensure that they were correctly made (Meacher, 1972). Cigarettes were not permitted within residents bedrooms or unsupervised (Meacher, 1972; Clough, 1981). Residents were not permitted to adjust the television or to possess knitting needles (Meacher, 1972). Residents were not permitted to go out alone (Meacher, 1972; Counsel and Care, 1992). More recently issues of surveillance have arisen including electronic tags, videos, intercoms and glass panels (Counsel and Care, 1992). Similarly the use of sedative drugs is also an issue (Meacher, 1972; Booth, 1985; Counsel and Care, 1992). Such availability of methods illustrates how the type of issue that arises and rationales that are provided may be affected by social development and economic factors at the time. Tea was provided only if residents walked to the dining room (Clough, 1981) and residents must get out of bed (Bolling Maynard et al, 1977). Margarine was provided, not butter (Clough, 1981). Such issues are not confined to Great Britain and are evident in other countries such as the USA (Tobin and Lieberman, 1976; Vladeck, 1980), and Australia (Newton, 1979), indicating the common existence of factors fundamental to caring and the need to identify them. There are also wider issues to consider; for example, the registration and inspection of nursing homes was proposed in 1905 finally occurring according to the Public Health Act 1936 (Townsend, 1964). The debate regarding who will fund places as well as who possess authority has been continuous. According to the Poor Law Commission 1930 all relatives were to be responsible; however, this was overturned by the National Assistance Act 1948 requiring local authorities to be responsible for the provision and funding of care but the spouse must also contribute to the funding (Means and Smith, 1983). Education of matrons and deputies was considered in 1949 but failed to occur due to staff shortages. The misplacement of residents into residential or nursing homes was recognised in 1950 (Means and Smith, 1983), halfway homes being proposed between the two which would involve moving a resident. Indeed the first home for the mentally ill was opened in the 1960s according to the Mental Health Act 1959 (Means and Smith, 1983). Alternatives to institutional care have historically been considered, such as reconsidering the size of homes, which ranged between 35 and 60 between 1948 and 1960 (Townsend, 1964); single rooms and group living also were considered in addition to community care (Townsend, 1964). Indeed what to call such homes has historically been a dilemma, suggestions including hostels or hotels (Means and Smith, 1983). The definition of long-term care is therefore largely socio-politically defined and how and where to care for such needy individuals has always been a dilemma. Issues cannot be divorced from historical events such as war because they affect predominant thoughts and priorities at the time. Whilst no nursing home is alike nor were all workhouses; care observed by the author includes routine bed, meal, drink, toilet times, restricted freedom for example:

- outings,

- smoking,

- alcohol,

- lack of physiotherapy or occupational therapy,

- use of rewards such as cigarettes,

reduced facilities, for example:

- flannels, gloves, and incontinence wipes,

- separation of husband and wife,

- discouragement of sexual relationships,

- lack of provision of personal facilities such as own tea making facilities or door keys.

Hence issues that arose within workhouses continue to arise today. In general there is evidence of staff division, staff control of residents, routine and hence reduced autonomy of residents. Indeed physical abuse is present within some (UKCC, 1994). What are the reasons for such actions or is it purely automatic? Such a service is no longer considered as a deterrent as were workhouses unless it is to deter reliance upon local authority funds since although community care is preferable, it may actually be less expensive. However, numerous rationales are provided as will be discussed.

5 DECISION MAKING

An individual may make numerous responses to a situation and select how to react directed by personal values and experiences (McGrew, 1982). Whether or not this is acted upon may depend upon sociological factors and an expected or desired mode of behaviour depending upon the individual's personal philosophy. Selected response is unassisted by lack of an aim of long-term care and lack of a general philosophy. All situations demand decision making. Individuals may however be unaware of utilising the decision-making process or reluctant to do so, thus promoting routine and the general application of decisions. The decision-making ability of the individual may also be restricted by bureaucracy which demands adherence to rules and regulations (Douglass RM, 1992).

A caring decision demands consideration of all possible alternative actions and consequences. As research increases, the variety of possible responses increases. Whether or not action is research based depends largely upon nurses' or care assistants' knowledge as well as residents' agreement to treatment. However, some actions in caring are not referred to by research, for example smoking unsupervised or trips out. This is possibly due to lack of recognition or awareness of such dilemmas and the necessary skills of the nurse, as well as lack of funds. The author is not suggesting that all actions be based upon research but survey research would highlight practice commonalities thus promoting more effective decision making. Such situations may be everyday issues. The nurse may even be unaware of possible alternatives and thus it may be unrecognisable as an issue. Nurses must be creative and flexible in order to respond to the individual resident or situation thus promoting quality of life of that resident. 'Quality of life refers to the ability to live one's own life according to one's own plan' (Young and Longman in

Goodinson and Singleton, 1984). A prime factor of this is autonomy of the resident or ability to make his or her own decisions, this being the degree to which one is human (Kant in Downie and Calman, 1987). Whilst a resident may not initially have planned to enter a nursing home there is no reason why he or she cannot adhere to his or her own life plan as far as possible. According to the Human Rights Act (1998) the needs and wishes of the individual must be maintained. Indeed, there are benefits to a resident controlling his or her own life (Chang, 1979), such as increased morale. Loss of control may actually hasten death (Dubree and Vogehlpohl, 1980). Relatives do not have the right to decide on behalf of the resident (Mason and McCall Smith, 1994). However, power of attorney gives a person decision-making capacity re finances. There is also a continuing power of attorney for those individuals with mental incapacity (Law Commission, 1979). Mental capacity is difficult to determine, yet some guidelines are available (Law Society and BMJ, 1995). Individuals may state what treatment they do or do not want in an advanced directive or living will (Haas, 2005). This is only used when the individual is unable to make decisions and must have been decided by the individual who was over 18 years old and had mental capacity at the time. At present, they are rarely used in the UK (Butterworth, 2005).

There will be a Mental Capacity Act in 2007 for England and Wales addressing the decision-making of individuals with mental illness (Age Concern, 2005). This will refer to decisions other than financial. In Scotland the Adults with Incapacity (Scotland) Act 2000 applies.

Decisions referring to medical treatment may be opposed according to the Mental Health Act (1983). Quality of the working life of staff may also be increased by promotion of residents' autonomy. However, some nurses do require guidance, for example the young or newly qualified. If so, they must recognise when decisions need making and refer to the more senior person. There are some individuals who prefer to control other individuals (Burger, 1989) or adopt the paternalistic approach (Agich, 1993) thus deciding for them. Whilst there may be various reasons for these situations occurring, the aim of this book is to offer a challenge to nurses and care staff by exploring all aspects of the issue.

These chapters shall identify some common issues that the author has observed within some care homes. The examples shall not be personalised other than by pseudonym to avoid detraction from the actual issue which may occur regardless of the age or condition of the individual concerned.

6 DECISIONS REGARDING INITIAL ENTRY TO A HOME

An individual should have maximum choice of which home to live in (National Assistance Act, 1948; Care Standards Act, 2000); however, this choice is often restricted. The restricting factors include: lack of awareness of other homes or the variation between them; lack of ability to visit them, possibly due to lack of transport; emergency admission; the availability of a bed and the home managers' willingness to accept the individual affected by factors such as the degree of dependency, for example.

Personal factors such as whether or not the home accepts people who smoke or pets may limit the choice of home. Choice of locality may be restricted due to the availability of homes within that area. There is, for example, a greater number of private homes within coastal areas, as there has historically been (Townsend, 1964), although this may be reduced by the redistribution of government funds according to the number of elderly per area (Laing and Buisson, 1994).

An individual may be unaware that he or she is going to a home or may be excluded from selection (Meacher, 1972; Wilcocks et al, 1987). Leaving their home is not an easy decision to make, especially if it harbours many memories, having lived there for most of their lives. Also to make new friends at this time of life is a huge expectation. To leave the home against their own volition may accelerate the process of institutionalisation and accompanying depression and hopelessness. Death of an individual may also be hastened by such a move (Tobin and Lieberman, 1976). Indeed, the effects of institutionalisation have been found to exist before admission to a home (Tobin and Lieberman, 1976). Choice may be further restricted by the use of block contracts by some local authorities, which involves the referral of residents to only those homes with a contract. This may have advantages for the home since residents will be automatically referred to them but they have additional requirements to adhere to. Such requirements may promote a quality service but it may be two-tier and the requirements should be applicable to all homes since they all have the same ultimate aim. However, such contracts may become obsolete since there is no government guidance for them and few local authorities use them (Laing, 1994).

There are businesses that will assist individuals with the selection of a home for a fee. Local authorities are not permitted to recommend certain ones. Some authorities do produce a list of guidelines to be used when assessing a home and Age Concern also provides advice.

The nurse may well be aware of a resident who has not been offered a choice. To mention alternatives may create further distress but if, following all attempts, the resident remains unsettled and unhappy, this should be further explored. However, the resident may choose to remain there rather than suffer the distress of moving again.

Mr Salmon is a young physically disabled resident and lives in a home amongst elderly individuals. He is unhappy and wishes to be moved to a home for the young physically disabled. What can the nurse do?

In this situation, the resident has clearly been misplaced and is not receiving appropriate care. It must be very depressing for somebody to live amongst so many elderly individuals certainly if his or her mind remains very active. He or she will have different occupational needs for example from the majority of residents and it will therefore be difficult for the staff to fulfil them. The nurse should question why the resident was placed there in the first place.

A number of young physically disabled individuals do actually remain within homes for older people due to a lack of provision of alternatives (Means and Smith, 1983). It may be very demoralising for the younger individual; however, it may create a more normal environment and some elderly individuals are extremely young in mind thus they may motivate and assist one another. This no longer occurs since April 2000 with the introduction of the Care Standards Act since homes cannot now admit residents whose needs they are unable to meet. A full assessment must be done before admission. However, it is included here as the situation may still exist. Indeed, there have been a number of residents who require nursing care, waiting in residential homes to be reassessed by social workers. These assessments are often delayed due to lack of funding (Nazarko, 1999).

If reassessment is taking a long time, this situation is a difficult one for the nurse to fight alone. He or she may have to refer to bodies such as the inspection team or Primary Care Trust and other agencies such as Age Concern who will offer much support and advice. The home owner or manager may be reluctant to refer the resident for another assessment because this may leave them with an empty bed. However, residents are entitled to be assessed again.

Mr and Mrs Sild live within a residential home but the physical condition of Mr Sild has deteriorated and he must now be transferred to a nursing home. This, however, means that both residents must be separated. Such enforced separation is inhuman. Indeed, the couple may have spent the majority of their lives together. Whether they have been married for a long time or not they still have a right to continue living together. Such separations are enforced according to the Registration of Nursing Homes Act (1984) and now the Care Standards Act (2000). However, if an individual becomes ill for a short length of time within a residential home, the district nurse may provide care. Each situation must be assessed upon an individual basis. Perhaps the district nurse could provide care in this situation? The proposed merger of nursing and residential homes may prevent such situations from occurring (Johnson and Hoyes, 2005) but it may well create additional problems.

Mrs Peacock wishes to continue living alone at home. However, the nurse is concerned about her unkempt condition and the filthy condition of the house. She may actually be compulsorily admitted to a nursing or residential home according to section 47 of the National Assistance Act (1948) although this applies for only three months before re-application is required (Freeman and Lyon, 1984). This should be a last resort for obvious reasons including the effect upon the individual. Whilst all individuals react differently, entering long-term care is rather traumatic anyway as previously discussed. Indeed this Act is rarely used for this purpose, about 200 times a year (Griffiths *et al*, 1990). Application to a magistrate's court must be made by a local community physician and local authority. Alternatively somebody may be admitted according to the Mental Health Act but must be registered as being mentally ill. Nurses and other professionals involved must examine their reasons for wishing the individual's removal to a home. For example, staff may be protecting themselves, fearing litigation should anything untoward occur whilst he or she is living alone at home. They may also desire to actually do something but they may do more by supporting him or her to live at home. There are other alternatives to be considered before taking such action. The individual may not be receiving the full amount of community services that he or she is entitled to, such as meals on wheels, and there may be various reasons for this. Perhaps he or she objects to contributing to the cost of such care or objects to having strangers in the house. Possibly a neighbour could have the key for use in emergencies. Indeed, guardianship may be used requiring attendance at a certain place such as a day centre, giving the guardian the right of access to that person (McPherson, 1988). However, it cannot be used to enforce entry and is only applicable if the individual is certified as being mentally ill. The individual may be happy as he or she is and may not endanger anybody else such as leaving the gas on, and to move them may actually reduce his or her quality of life.

There are a high number of individuals in care homes suffering from dementia (Bruce *et al*, 2002). Whilst currently there are some homes for the elderly mentally ill, the accommodation of confused individuals amongst non-confused, continues. Indeed individuals who are not confused may be misplaced into a home for the elderly mentally ill. Separation of the elderly mentally ill may ensure the provision of a more specialised and safe environment (Goodwin, 1993).

Decisions regarding initial entry to the home

It may also promote a more peaceful environment for residents who are not confused since confused residents may wander into their room or shout. Whilst either situation is difficult for the nurse, it requires nurses who possess special skills to be able to care for residents within a home for the elderly mentally ill and as such, they will require additional support. Individuals who are so confused may also have the same degree of physical disability as other individuals. Therefore the nurse must possess skills in all areas of care. However, in some districts, regulations only require qualified nurses within such homes to be registered as a Registered Mental Nurse (RMN). Alternatively, the provision of a more mixed environment may maintain stimulation for the residents and it may be stigmatising to separate them.

7 DECISIONS REGARDING OUTINGS

Mr Greenwood is 82 and walks with a stick. He wishes to go out alone. What action could be taken?

1. Forbid or dissuade him from going out;
2. Restrain him;
3. Accompany him there and back;
4. Follow him unbeknown to him.

The nurse may argue that he may be knocked down or become drunk if going to the pub or catch a cold if it is poor weather. Mr Greenwood may indeed be knocked down as we all may be but prefer to risk his life by crossing a road, as he would do if he lived at home alone. Need he inform the nurse where he is going at all? Whilst this is advisable regarding fire procedures, indeed homes are required to have a signing in and out book, isn't this some form of restriction of freedom? However, if he refuses to abide by this rule the home manager is within his rights to refuse to accommodate him. The nurse may worry that he may catch cold but if he wraps up well and the nurse can prove that full advice has been given, it is Mr Greenwood's decision.

Legally a nurse cannot prevent a resident going out alone unless of course according to section 2 of the Mental Health Act 1983; but then dilemmas arise regarding the definition of mentally ill although one or more doctors are involved in the diagnosis depending upon which section of the act is involved. This Act does not apply, however, to individuals suffering from dementia, for example (Bennet and Kingston, 1993). Even if mobile only within a wheelchair the individual possesses the same rights as everybody else. There are also advocacy groups particularly for the mentally ill and disabled who may contribute towards such decisions (Appendix 1). If in the nurse's opinion the resident is extremely confused and unsafe out alone, the police and social worker must be involved. If the resident does go out alone, the police may find the resident and encourage a review. It is illegal to enforce a resident to return or to restrain a resident in order to prevent wandering (Young, 1992). However, diversions may be attempted. If the home is for the mentally ill, the majority of residents may tend to wander. Therefore ethics are questioned regarding the use of top and bottom door handles, video cameras and tagging, all of which are a form of restraint (Counsel and Care, 1992), but isn't observing a resident a form of restraint?

Whilst there are no recorded court cases of residents suing for false imprisonment (Griffiths *et al*, 1990) there are cases regarding residents being killed or injured due to going out alone (Norman, 1980). Individuals may not be in a position to initiate court intervention due to cost, ability, knowledge or lack of witnesses but they are within their rights to do so.

If a member of staff accompanies him there and returns to collect him, similar arguments ensue and it is rather like nursery care of children. So too is secretly following him as well as betraying his trust and invading his privacy.

Alternatively, a full assessment of Mr Greenwood's capabilities, desires and needs, could have been undertaken, action and outcome being recorded within the care plan and on a risk assessment. The nurse may be protected even more so if countersigned by the resident or his advocate since the care plan is potentially a legal document.

Conversely, Mr Dale is 86 and does not wish to go on the day trip with seven other residents. What action could the nurse take?

1. Force him onto the bus and insist that he will enjoy it when he arrives;
2. Abide by Mr Dale's decision;
3. Offer Mr Dale trips alone.

It is possible that Mr Dale may enjoy it when he arrives. However, he has decided not to go. Whose needs would be satisfied by enforcing him to go? Would the nurse have felt comfortable to prescribe such action upon the nursing records?

It may be an indication of the parent role with the nurse attending to the resident as a child, possibly to fulfil his or her own needs. It may be some form of extreme rehabilitation. However, by removing the choice from the individual, rehabilitation is not being achieved, only submission. To force Mr Dale onto the bus would be assault (Dimond, 2002), as would be touching an individual if he or she does not desire it.

If the nurse abides by Mr Dale's decision without fully exploring or attempting to explore reasons, the nurse is not fulfilling his or her role. It is, however, the nurse's role to advise and not to insist. Insisting is the antithesis of caring since it is done only to achieve the aims as perceived by the carer, not the one being cared for. This is paternalism. It is necessary with children who are too young to be aware of possible outcomes and who have yet to learn. However, the elderly have lived the majority of their lives learning from past experience and establishing personal values. It is the nurse's role to assess this. One must be cruel to be kind, they say, but what are we achieving?

Trips could be offered alone but it is essential that the nurse fully assesses Mr Dale before considering action. There may be some other reason for his refusal to go on the trip. Assumptions may promote inappropriate care. Ultimately, it is ethically and morally the resident's decision. There may be circumstances when the resident is rather depressed and the nurse considers that going out would reduce depression. Again this is the nurse's perception only. What is really being gained? To oppose the resident's own choice, thus reducing self-control of his life, may create depression (Dubree and Vogehlpohl, 1980).

Wheelchairs

According to a district policy new residents within care homes are not provided with an individual wheelchair unless they sit in it all day. Wheelchairs are only provided for individuals (Nazarko, 1995). Whilst wheelchairs may be hired it is the responsibility of the home owner to purchase a transit chair; wheelchairs are consequently not properly looked after and residents are unable to go out.

Decisions regarding residents outings

It is the responsibility of the home manager to ensure that such wheelchairs are bought or hired and to take further action if this is not the case.

Again, in addition to monitoring the situation the identification of a separate problem within the care plan would be of benefit. For example, 'Mr Adams is unable to go out because – .' Perhaps the District Authority is unaware of the effect of this policy on the residents.

8 DECISIONS REGARDING EATING

Mrs Black is an 80-year-old obese lady but she enjoys her food and is reluctant to commence a diet. What could the nurse do?

1. Insist upon it;
2. Involve the doctor, dietician, Mrs Black and/or her advocate;
3. Offer healthy options;
4. Encourage Mrs Black to join a weight-reducing group or form one for the home.

The nurse may argue that staff may damage their backs when lifting her or Mrs Black may develop a heart condition. The nurse's reluctance to take risks is evident; if Mrs Black's health worsens there may be an inquiry thus: 'Why wasn't Mrs Black having a reducing diet?' Use of lifting aids and correct technique should reduce concern of the nurses harming their backs. Whilst a high quality of working life must be maintained – hopefully to reflect upon care practice – how much weight is an 80-year-old person really going to lose? How many additional years of life is she going to gain? How many does she want? Again another conflict between nurse and resident is illustrated. Residents may aim for quality of life meaning they would rather achieve satisfaction of their desires. Nurses may aim for quantity of life meaning residents would hopefully live longer and be physically healthier, based upon the medical model of care. However, evidence indicates that a reduction in quality of life may actually inadvertently affect health and thus quantity of life, for example by causing depression (Tobin and Lieberman, 1976). This may also possess monetary implications for treatment such as drugs but this ought not to be the sole reason for promoting quality of life as will be illustrated.

Commencing a diet regardless of a resident's wishes is

equivalent to the withholding of food. This may be avoided by the second alternative of involving other relevant people such as dieticians. However, they are not permitted to overrule a resident's decision either, so hopefully Mrs Black or her advocate would also be involved.

A wide healthy choice of food could be offered at all times but must not replace the resident's usual choice or preference. A full assessment of Mrs Black must be undertaken identifying needs, desires, alternatives and interests. Possibly Mrs Black is suffering from boredom for example. Ultimately she may only be advised. This must be documented as a problem in the care plan. If the resident does not agree with a diet, then records could be made of how the nurse has encouraged her but that she has refused treatment.

Similarly Mr Ball is diabetic and secretly eats sweets or demands puddings. Hence there may be a constant battle between nurse and resident. In this case the nurse could:

1. Remove the sweets from Mr Ball;
2. Discuss with Mr Ball and his relatives, advising them not to bring him sweets;
3. Involve the doctor and dietician;
4. Contact the diabetic association.

To remove the sweets from Mr Ball would be theft. Mr Ball, and his relatives if they are involved, must certainly be spoken to before any action is taken. However, they may only be advised; to insist that Mr Ball does not eat sweets would be enforcing medical treatment. Perhaps Mr Ball would be happy for the staff to keep his sweets for him, thus monitoring his intake. This would be an acceptable approach if Mr Ball was happy about it but it may remove some of the enjoyment of eating the sweets. Again the nurse could not insist upon this action. Indeed Mr Ball may ask one of the staff to bring sweets in for him. If the carer refuses she risks damaging her relationship with Mr Ball. If she agrees to do so, she risks opposing her contract of employment. However, does she enforce the medical treatment by refusing to fetch him sweets or does she adhere to Mr Ball's wishes thus maintaining his quality of life?

If the doctor was contacted it would legally protect the nurse who can then prove that action had been taken. The doctor may also assess Mr Ball for possible sugar imbalances. He may for example be suffering from episodes of hypoglycaemia unless he just enjoys sweets. The diabetic association may also be of value, providing Mr Ball with further information and motivation.

Puddings made with diabetic sugar could be offered. Indeed, some homes may make all puddings with diabetic sugar anyway but then that is restricting the choice of individuals who are not diabetic. Does the nurse have the right not to give Mr Ball a pudding if he requests it? If the nurse provides food containing sugar at his request, it may be deemed mild euthanasia; whilst it may not be for that purpose, it may ultimately contribute towards the acceleration of Mr Ball's death; hence the fear of some nurses! Both of the latter examples involve residents' refusal to adhere to nursing or medical treatment. Legally treatment cannot be enforced in opposition to an individual's consent. This does not mean, however, that nurses must automatically abide by residents' wishes. In order to choose residents require appropriate knowledge. It is the nurse's role to provide this advice where it is lacking. Therefore if the nurse records that this has been done, within the nursing records, the nurse is legally protected. This does not mean that the case may not reach the courts.

From a moral or ethical aspect, would the nurse feel comfortable opposing the resident's desires? This may depend upon the nurse's own values as well as the resident's. As discussed, the nurse may aim for quantity of life considering the needs of the resident, from the nurse's perception, that must be fulfilled. Since the resident does not desire to adhere to a diet thus aiming for quality of life, it is not a personal need for him. Hence there is a difference between needs and desires.

Similarly Mr Duckham has a condition requiring a low fat diet. He refuses to adhere to the diet, refusing all low fat alternatives and constantly requesting ordinary meals from the nurse. In this case, the nurse and resident must speak to the doctor. Ultimately ordinary meals must be provided to prevent starvation. It must also be documented in the care plan that Mr Duckham will not adhere to the diet and the attempts the nurse has made to encourage him.

All residents are provided with skimmed milk and margarine instead of butter because it is considered to be healthier for them. However, after so many years of taking milk and butter this will reduce the residents' quality of life since they are not being permitted to adhere to their usual choice. There may also be monetary implications for the home since margarine is cheaper than butter but skimmed milk is slightly more expensive thus erasing this as a rationale. What is going to be achieved by this so late in life? What right have staff to alter such things without first asking the residents?

At mealtimes some residents would like to have personal use of condiments, butter, jam and teapots. What could the nurse do?

1. Forbid it;
2. Allow some residents to use them;
3. Assess each resident on an individual basis for their capabilities and desire.

If the nurse forbids such independence it echoes the treatment of young children and is therefore infantalisation. The nurse may argue that residents may apply 'too much' regarding condiments such as vinegar; they may apply it inappropriately to the wrong food, or they may burn themselves upon the teapots. Individual assessments are essential as well as risk assessments, in order to assess a resident's physical and psychological capabilities as well as desire. Mrs Red may not even desire to have such independence hence the nurse must guard against imposing it upon her. Inclusion of others, such as the doctor or occupational therapist, in such an assessment would strengthen the conclusion and they may suggest alternative means of making it possible. However, if a resident still insists when he or she is not deemed to be capable, what then? Residents must be supervised if a difficulty is suspected and this may be done less obviously, from a distance.

It may be argued that insufficient time is available. Such considerations are, however, one aspect of caring. It may be possible to re-organise mealtimes, which may involve rescheduling of other activities such as break times, and you never know until you try.

Mr Rose is 78 years old and he commented that he would like fish and chips from the fish shop or jam roly-poly occasionally. As nurses it is our aim within long-term care to ensure that such desires are fulfilled. Some nurses may argue that everybody would want fish and chips and not all would be able to afford it. Surely some arrangement could be made? Not all residents may want them but if they do what about some fund-raising if the manager cannot provide? Why should Mr Rose be deprived on behalf of the majority? Aren't there occasions when you have something that your friends could not afford? This is a fact of everyday life. Life within a nursing home is not within a sterile environment. The kitchen staff may argue that it would be inconvenient to cook jam roly-poly or residents' preferences since they have a fortnightly menu rota. Whilst good relations are essential between the kitchen staff, nurses and budget holders, promoted by discussion and involvement, it is not necessarily more expensive or harder work.

Mr Gresham is 84 and requests to eat his dinner within his bedroom, not in the dining room with the other residents. What could the nurse do?

1. Physically enforce him to come out of his room;
2. Mislead him into coming out of his room;
3. Advise him to go out of his room;
4. Permit him to remain in his room.

The nurse fears that he will never come out of his room otherwise or may become depressed. The nurse also regards coming out of his room as a form of rehabilitation.

If the nurse enforced Mr Gresham to come out of his room by bodily moving him, this is abuse. Indeed, he would probably be so upset afterwards that he would not eat anything anyway. The nurse could mislead him by saying that his room needs cleaning so he has to come out anyway but such manipulation is a form of abuse since it directly opposes Mr Gresham's choice.

There may be additional reasons of staff inconvenience

since it may take more time to provide meals for residents within their rooms, certainly if a large number require it. However, it may not be impossible if all staff are involved and aware of what is occurring. Where meals are eaten is an important factor regarding nutritional intake since, as discussed, it may deter Mr Gresham from eating. Hence it is important to assess him in order to identify why he does not wish to come out of his room. He may, for example, dislike eating amongst 40 other residents all the time since he has eaten on his own for the last 20 years. He may not like the residents he sits next to at the dinner table or it may be very noisy there. He may be feeling a little depressed and desire his own company that day. Individuals do not feel the same all of the time therefore they may vary their routine accordingly. He may just prefer to be alone anyway or he may be trying to regain self-control by opposing what his instructions are.

Whose needs would be met by enforcing Mr Gresham to come out of his room? How many of us really live amongst so many other people and like the company of others all of the time? We must examine the true rationale for our actions in order to meet the needs of the individual effectively.

Mrs Grey is 90 and will not feed herself. Whilst she is able to feed herself with effort she would rather be fed by a nurse.

What could the nurse do?

1. Refuse to feed her arguing that she must maintain her independence;
2. Feed her;
3. Provide finger foods that she need not use utensils for.

If the nurse refuses to feed her, Mrs Grey may not have any dinner hence it is the equivalent of depriving her of food. It is also failure to provide appropriate care since, for whatever reason, Mrs Grey is not feeding herself. Possible reasons for her failure to feed herself must be explored involving other professionals such as the doctor. She may suffer from painful wrists or require adaptations such as a plate guard for example. It is suggested that Mrs Grey has observed other residents being fed and requires to be similarly attended to. This would obviously signify an unmet need of Mrs Grey.

Perhaps she needs the nurses' attention, feeling lonely for example. Indeed, nurses may communicate more with residents when undertaking such tasks for them. Mrs Grey could be fed initially but, with encouragement, she may be motivated to feed herself eventually. This differs from the refusal of food since Mrs Grey eats when fed. However, the nurse could alternatively be accused of professional negligence due to the withholding of food, especially since it may harm Mrs Grey's health. The fact that Mrs Grey will not feed herself must be documented as a problem so the nurse can indicate what has been done about it.

Mr Brown requests a cup of tea but it is not drinks time yet. The nurse may refuse to give him one explaining that it is not drinks time yet and if he has one everybody will want one. This again is the equivalent of withholding food. It is the nurse's role to provide him with such care. However, does the nurse's role require her to provide only sufficient food or drink and if so from whose perspective? If a resident requests a drink there is obviously a need for one. Perhaps Mr Brown likes tea or is simply bored. The nurse may be busy but surely somebody is not too busy to make a cup of tea? If they are, staff numbers require reviewing. A small kitchen may be of benefit. Perhaps Mr Brown and some residents may be capable of making their own tea – but that is another issue. Volunteers would also be beneficial. Alternatively drinks such as orange juice could be left available. It may also have cost implications and that requires discussion with the administrator. If alternative drinks are left available it is argued that they may be knocked over or if not diabetic orange juice, a diabetic resident would drink some. Whilst such drinks should be left within the residents' rooms, not all possess a key and some residents share a room. Such drinks should be freshly made daily and kept within a covered jug. Ultimately it may be easier to prepare a drink for a resident as and when requested. Indeed, this also enables him or her to exercise self-control by requesting something.

Mrs Stamp is 80, has difficulty swallowing and tends to choke on her food.

What could the nurse do?

Decisions regarding eating

1. Provide liquidised meals;
2. Cut food up very small and supervise Mrs Stamp when eating.

Providing such soft diets limits Mrs Stamp's choice of food. Mealtimes may be the highlight of Mrs Stamp's day, not just a physical necessity. There should always be an alternative choice available to prevent the frequent provision of mashed potato and mince. Why not liquidise what she would like and keep it in separate portions? Often liquidised meals are liquidised together like porridge which looks very unappetising. There may be some occasions when Mrs Stamp may not require liquidised food and the nurse may not know this until she has attempted it.

Before doing anything, a full assessment must be made involving the dietician. However, dietician referrals take a long time in a care home. A problem must be noted in the care plan and a risk assessment done.

Cases involving choking have, in the past, reached the courts. If the nurse is aware of the possibility of choking, he or she must be prepared to illustrate what precautions were taken. Of course a resident may help him or herself to another's food. Whilst this may be an example of the refusal of treatment if it is proven that the resident is of sound mind, actions must be taken to avoid this within the immediate area of the resident, certainly if the nurse is aware of such a tendency. Of course it may also be an indication of hunger!

Mrs Ardine is 78 and wishes to wash up in the kitchen. What could the nurse do?

1. Forbid it;
2. Permit it;
3. Supervise her;
4. Assess her individually, involving GP, registration officer, advocate, and discuss with health and safety officers.

Matron may be concerned about health and safety regulations. Whilst there is a need for such regulations, surely there is an alternative? Indeed, children within residential homes should be encouraged to assist with meals or make snacks and drinks according to the Children Act 1989. However, the children should be supervised if necessary and within a large home it may be necessary to provide a small cooking area away from the main kitchen. Similarly, children are encouraged to do their own laundry, again with separate facilities if necessary; then why not the elderly? Health and safety regulations require white coats to be worn in the kitchen, hands to be washed and a temperature of 50–60 degrees for washing up water (Health and Safety Executive, 1993). Some homes do have small kitchens for residents' use; however, not all homes have this advantage. Surely residents could wash their hands and wear the appropriate attire as do kitchen staff? Indeed, there is a recorded case of some residents successfully winning a court battle regarding this and being permitted to make tea without wearing overalls; however, they must be worn when cooking. The kitchen staff must be considered. Although it may be inappropriate to permit residents in the kitchen whilst the general meals are being cooked perhaps they could bake buns or make themselves a cup of tea under supervision. Washing up of cups or even medicine pots could be undertaken outside the kitchen in a bowl. If this does oppose regulations it could always be washed later in the usual way.

Mr Scarf is 78 years old and would like an alcoholic drink. However, he regularly takes sedatives as prescribed. What could the nurse do?

Again there is a conflict between quality and quantity of life. It is necessary to consider the individual's case, for example, the state of his health and possibility of it improving. Even if it could improve, the decision is ultimately the individual's, both legally and morally. However, the nurse is the one who provides or permits alcohol, rather like sugary food to a diabetic. The doctor should be consulted, certainly if Mr Scarf is a heavy drinker. Alcohol may even be prescribed but there should be no need to do this and it erases the purpose of drinking for sheer pleasure. Some nursing homes may not permit alcohol at all, certainly not within residents' cupboards. It may be argued that other residents may take the alcohol – all the more reason to provide locker keys. Why shouldn't residents be allowed to drink as much as they desire at their leisure? They could be informed of the potential harm and it is essential to make full records within the nursing care plan.

An additional rationale for forbidding Mr Scarf to drink may be to prevent drunkenness. However, such vibes are part of everyday life, of being alive, for some people.

9 DECISIONS REGARDING HEALTH CARE

Mr Crown will not permit the nurse to contact the doctor and it is indicated that medical treatment may be needed. If Mr Crown had dementia, it would need to be a team decision involving relatives. Individuals with dementia have a right to make decisions also. What could the nurse do?

To inform the doctor against the resident's wishes would oppose the confidentiality of the resident but not to do so may harm the resident.

The nurse must explain to the resident that a doctor is necessary and record this within the care plan. Indeed, there may be some reason why the resident does not wish to see the doctor such as fear. The resident's relatives or friends may also be able to help provided that the resident wishes them to be informed.

Ultimately the nurse must contact the doctor and whether or not the resident will see the doctor is up to the resident. The home manager may indeed decide not to care for the resident on this basis.

Conversely, a resident may insist that the nurse contact the doctor even though the nurse does not think that it is necessary.

The nurse must discuss this further with the resident and record the action and outcome within the care plan. There may be some reason for this, for example loneliness or symptoms that the resident has not reported to the nurse. Ultimately the nurse must contact the doctor, who may speak to the resident further if the visit was unnecessary, particularly if it is a regular occurrence.

Medication

Mr Faulds refuses to take his tablets.
What could the nurse do?

1. Enforce him to take the medication;
2. Hide the medication in food or drink;
3. Split the capsule or crush the tablet.

To enforce the medication would be abuse (Brazier, 1992) even if Mr Faulds suffers from dementia. Yet hiding medication in food is common practice within nursing homes (Duffin, 2000). Guidelines state that medication may be added to food or drink when the individual lacks capacity to refuse it and with documented team agreement (UKCC, 2001; Royal Pharmaceutical Society, 2003). However, the difficulty is determining the capacity of individuals, although there are guidelines, as discussed earlier.

Splitting capsules or crushing tablets is also common practice in nursing but by doing this, the nurse risks harming the resident (James, 2004). It thus opposes the NMC code of conduct which states 'You must act to identify and minimise risk to patients and clients'.

Residents do have the right to refuse treatment. There have been disciplinary cases regarding the enforced administration of medication by nurses (UKCC, 1994).

The reason for the nurse's insistence must be acknowledged. Would Mr Faulds survive without these tablets or are they administered for the benefit of staff and other residents? This would be a form of restraint. Brooks speaks strongly, but correctly, of chemical straitjacketing (Fry, 1992).

If somebody will not take their medication, the nurse must offer all encouragement. This ensures that it is an informed choice (Young, 1992) as well as indicating that the nurse has taken appropriate action. Possible reasons must be considered. Perhaps Mr Faulds feels that the tablet is difficult to swallow. If so, liquids can be obtained. Boots the Chemist are able to manufacture any medication in a liquid form. However the cost may be too great for the doctor. The doctor must be informed of a refusal to take medication, and relatives too if the resident wishes. A problem must be documented in the care plan indicating what has been done about it.

Mrs Gibbard wishes to keep and take her own tablets. However the nurse will not permit it, stating that the tablets may be lost or taken by other residents or be taken incorrectly.

According to the Care Standards 2003, residents are now to be encouraged to self-medicate. A locked cupboard must be kept within Mrs Gibbard's room which may also be locked. Indeed children older than 16 within residential care may keep and take their own medication (Children's Act 1989: HMSO, 1991). However, it is essential to undertake an individual assessment of Mrs Gibbard regarding her capabilities and needs. She may, for example, require readily prepared tablets in individual containers. Supervision may be required initially or she may need reminding. It should also be discussed with her GP. A medication card providing information regarding the drugs could be issued to Mrs Gibbard in a form that she is able to read and understand.

Medications that are taken as required are another issue. Mrs Gibbard may be permitted to keep such as paracetemol if she is unwilling to give them to the nurse and has been assessed as capable. The home manager could of course refuse to care for her on this basis. There are often residents who keep such medicines as paracetemol in their handbags. The nurse may only provide advice and record within the care plan and on a risk assessment, informing the doctor and other staff. To remove the medication against the resident's will would be stealing.

Mrs Atkin needs regular anti-epileptic drugs but refuses to take them. Even if Mrs Atkin was in the establishment according to section 2 of the Mental Health Act, such medications could not be enforced. Only treatment for the mental condition for which she has been sectioned may be so administered and, even then, strict conditions apply. This must be discussed with Mrs Atkin's doctor. If Mrs Atkin was within her own home her refusal to take the drugs may be unknown to others. The discussion with the doctor, its outcome and any attempts to encourage Mrs Atkin must be recorded within the care plan and her refusal to take tablets identified as a separate problem.

Decisions regarding health care

Mrs Smith's morning tablets are due but she is sleeping soundly. The nurse does not know whether or not to wake her up.

To wake Mrs Smith up may be regarded as invasion of her privacy. Not to wake her up when she has requested to be woken may be regarded as withholding medication.

This must be discussed with Mrs Smith's doctor and with Mrs Smith herself. Perhaps the drug administration times could be altered?

It is advisable to give medications that are required at specific times, for example, anti-Parkinson's drugs or some antibiotics. However, Mrs Smith may refuse to permit the nurse to wake her. This must be recorded within the care plan as a separate problem.

Mrs Everett is prescribed antibiotics which must be given four times a day at regular intervals. The tablet times are 6, 12, 6, 12 so that Mrs Everett is woken at midnight. It is the nurse who sets the tablet times but in order to ensure equal intervals of administration, Mrs Everett must be woken at some time during the night. Again, this is invasion of Mrs Everett's privacy, if she does not wish to be woken. There are very few individuals who would wake during the night for medication other than an essential drug. This must be discussed with Mrs Everett's doctor and the pharmacist to ascertain the importance of such regularity.

Pharmacology regulations pertaining to care homes are determined nationally and locally. Some areas possess a locally agreed list of remedies such as drapolene cream which may be applied for a certain length of time as homely remedy, prior to prescription. This practice is recommended (Royal Pharmaceutical Society of GB, 2003). If it is not adopted, nothing at all should be applied or administered without prescription. This may not assist situations at weekends or bank holidays, for example. From the author's experience, not all nurses or managers are aware of this. It is the nurse's responsibility to approach the district pharmacist for information regarding this. Medication or dressings should only be used for the resident for whom they are prescribed (Royal Pharmaceutical Society of GB, 2003).

Indwelling Therapy

Mrs Farmer is refusing to eat and drink. There may be many situations when this arises; for example, cerebro-vascular accidents or depression. The nurse considers that an intravenous infusion or nasogastric therapy may be necessary. However, does Mrs Farmer want such treatment? Is she likely to pull the tubes out? Does she actually require terminal care? This must be discussed with the care team and medical team with Mrs Farmer and her relatives if she wishes.

Mrs Farmer may desire to be left in peace. Indeed, what is really going to be gained by increasing the quantity of her life in this way? If Mrs Farmer does refuse treatment there may actually be reasons for this such as boredom or confusion hence all possibilities must be considered.

The nurse fears litigation due to Mrs Farmer's possible starvation or dehydration if no such treatment is commenced. Indeed, in America the courts did support the patient's rights to refuse treatment (Mason and Smith, 1994) but conversely, they opposed a 90-year-old patient's son's wishes not to commence nasogastric therapy (Fiesta, 1988).

If such treatment is in progress its removal may not be permitted. However, removal from a comatose patient has been supported (Fiesta, 1988) hence it depends very much upon individual circumstances and is not a decision that the doctor or nurse can make alone. A resident who is not comatose may make a request for the discontinuation of such treatment. Discontinuing treatment differs to commencing treatment and this would be a case for the courts.

If something can be done the doctor is obliged to provide treatment unless the resident refuses it. If the resident is unable to decide, because it is an emergency for example, the doctor must provide treatment as though it is desired. Relatives are not legally able to consent or refuse consent. Not to commence treatment would be the equivalent of passive euthanasia, more so if the resident is in agreement with it, or else manslaughter. Treatment may only be commenced in opposition to an individual's wishes according to section 2 of the Mental Health Act as previously discussed.

Decisions regarding health care

If there is little hope of recovery it may be preferable for the resident to remain within the home. However, some cases may be quickly reversed by infusions, for example diabetic coma, despite the resident's age. Hence it would be appropriate to provide hospital treatment before returning the resident home. Some care homes are able to provide care for residents with intravenous infusions or subcutaneous infusions. This is made more possible by the existence of crisis intervention teams within the community. Whilst these may be doctors' decisions, nurses have much influence upon doctors in such situations which are a major dilemma for the professions.

Certainly before considering such treatments, all other action should have been taken first. This includes such as commencing and maintaining food or fluid charts, offering small portions and spending time with the resident. A problem must also be identified in the care plan and the doctor informed at an early stage.

Similarly, there are debates concerning resuscitation (Mason and Smith, 1994). Generally all individuals must be resuscitated unless they have expressed a desire not to be resuscitated (Mason and Smith, 1994). This creates a dilemma when the resident suffers from a terminal illness or extreme dementia, for example. There may be a case for a living will which is accepted if written by an individual who had mental capacity at the time (Making Decisions Alliance, 2003). It is recommended that a resident be asked about their wishes regarding death and dying on admission (Care Standards, 2003) and the home should also have a policy regarding this. The dilemma for the nurse is when and how to ask the resident. The author recommends a small booklet tastefully presented that the resident, or relative if he or she wishes, may complete.

10 DECISIONS REGARDING RELIGIOUS NEEDS

Mr Trellone wishes to attend church every Sunday but there is not enough staff to accompany him or her and transport is unavailable. What could the nurse do?

Attending church is very important to some individuals especially if they have been a regular attender in the past. It also provides somewhere for the resident to go and regular contact with the outside community. It is the responsibility of the home manager to ensure that the residents' needs are met. Indeed, if such needs are not met the resident may be harmed; for example, depression may ensue due to reduced personal control as well as being unable to go out. This should be recorded as a problem within the resident's care plan and evaluated accordingly.

Possibly the home manager could ensure that an extra member of staff is available that day to take the resident to church. Home owners may be unable to pay for an extra member of staff so volunteers may be able to do this. The church could also be contacted and they may be able to collect and return the resident to the home. However, nurses may then be concerned about the resident going out without a member of staff.

There may some residents within the home who are unable to attend church due to a high level of dependency or they may be of a different religion that may not be provided for within the community, such as Moslem. In such cases, it would be preferable that a separate room is available for private prayer and the relevant religious person should be encouraged to attend.

Mrs Doe does not celebrate Christmas because she is a Jehovah's Witness. Most homes at Christmas are decorated

43

throughout and Father Christmas attends. Nurses must ensure that that is what the resident wants. Some residents may wish to be totally separate from such celebrations but must not remain forgotten within their room. Individual beliefs and values must be respected and understood at all times. Provision for residents' religious needs is a requirement of the care standards (Care Standards, 2003).

11 DECISIONS REGARDING WALKING

Mrs White is not provided with a wheelchair when she requests it and hence is forced to walk. This is illegal (Dimond, 2002).

The nurse must discover why Mrs White does not wish to walk. Has her sense of life's purpose diminished? If so, is it possible to rekindle it? Attempts must be made to identify what Mrs White's hobbies are. The nurse must communicate regularly with her and note which staff she has a good relationship with. Perhaps she is more likely to walk with them as well as her relatives if she has any. Short-term goals could be made with a landmark such as 'walk to the front door'.

Mrs White's health problems may interfere with her ability. These may include deafness, blindness or tiredness. The latter may be due to illnesses such as depression, diabetes or anaemia, or result from medication such as sedatives. A full assessment of, and with, Mrs White is essential regarding physical as well as psychological factors. Indeed, Mrs White may not regard her inability or reluctance to walk as a problem at all or is that the problem? This may only be discovered by an assessment which must be fully recorded within the care plan with the action and outcome. The nurse needs to document his or her efforts to address the problem.

Mr Watts walks very unsteadily, usually with a frame. However, he often attempts to climb the stairs. The nurses have therefore fitted a safety gate across the bottom of the stairway. This is a form of restraint and a potential fire and safety hazard; for example, residents may fall over it. This action thus endangers the majority in order to protect Mr Watts' physical safety. Indeed, any individual staff or resident or visitor is capable of falling downstairs. It also opposes Mr Watts' autonomy since he obviously wishes to go upstairs. Possible reasons for this must be explored thus indicating

45

possible methods by which the dilemma may be resolved. Mr Watts may be looking for the toilet, for example, which in his former house was situated upstairs. The nurse could observe Mr Watts when he walks, possibly walking with him if he or she permits it. Again, full records must be made within the nursing records indicating that nurses are aware of this and action has been taken. A risk assessment must also be completed for Mr Watts.

12 DECISIONS REGARDING RESTRAINT

Mrs Dix frequently stands up and falls. The nurse restrains her by fastening her to a chair around her waist. Staff are wondering whether or not to commence sedatives. Such action is a form of false imprisonment (Dimond, 2002), trespass or assault (Counsel and Care, 1992) and Mrs Dix or her advocate may take legal action. Restraint must only be used temporarily and when absolutely necessary to prevent injury to the resident or another person (Young, 1992).

The nurse is confronted by the problem and tries to solve it instantly by giving care to the resident. What about caring with Mrs Dix by obtaining an in-depth assessment involving her advocate or relatives if she has any, along with other team members? Mrs Dix may simply enjoy walking, for example. If so, a nurse could accompany her upon regular walks. Indeed, she may require to use the toilet or have previously been a very active lady. She may even wish to sit somewhere else. It may not be possible for a nurse to sit with her all the time – and even that is a form of restraint, but surely somebody could observe the area? She may also like some form of activity to undertake. Full records, including a risk assessment, must be made identifying the problem and the action taken.

Similarly, Mr Lake wanders out of bed during the night. If this is a frequent occurrence there is obviously a need for something but this should again be considered upon an individual basis. Call mats may be useful in some cases to alert the nurse. If bed sides are used there is the possibility that Mr Lake may climb over them. Indeed, there have been court cases regarding this (Ramprogus and Gibson, 1991). There have also been court cases regarding the failure to use bed sides (Kapp in Agich, 1993).

The use of bed sides must thus be very carefully considered

following discussions with the doctor. A risk assessment must be done (MDA, 2001) and a problem identified in the care plan. Indeed, some homes use disclaimers. If bed sides are used, a consent form could be signed by the resident or relative but the legality of this is questionable. It does not prove that informed consent has been given and relatives cannot legally consent (Mason and McCall Smith, 1994).Nor is it legal to opt out of responsibility if injury or death has occurred (Dimond, 2005) according to the Unfair Contract Terms Act (1977).

A mattress placed upon the floor may soften the landing should Mr Lake fall. Whilst it may not look very professional and may hinder nursing staffs' lifting technique it will serve its purpose. Any visitors must be informed, however, to prevent misunderstandings.

Mr Johns frequently removes his dressings. His hands are bound with bandages and loosely tied to the bed sides when in bed. This is restraint, assault and a form of abuse. Mr Johns may take civil action against the nurse.

Again the full situation must be assessed. The dressings may irritate Mr Johns, for example, or he may be unaware of the importance of them. Perhaps there is an alternative dressing that may suit him? His doctor may also emphasise the importance of dressings as would his relatives if he has any. It may help if he has more to occupy him during the day. Perhaps a nurse could sit with him and talk to him. This is similar to Mr Johns refusing treatment and it is his right to do so. Again, all actions and outcomes must be recorded within the nursing care plan.

Mrs Hunter was a very confused lady who constantly wandered. She never slept at night hence she was commenced upon night sedation following a nurse's suggestion to the doctor.

A full assessment of Mrs Hunter would have revealed possible underlying reasons; for example she may have felt cold or hungry or been looking for the toilet. Indeed, she may have been looking for her own bed at home, certainly if only recently admitted.

This may have been Mrs Hunter's usual sleep pattern, hence the importance of undertaking an assessment upon admission involving relatives if possible. Less sleep is required by the elderly anyway (Wilson, 2003).

The ethics of administering tablets to Mrs Hunter without her knowledge is also questionable since consent has not therefore been obtained for treatment. Ever heard the nurse who replies this is a vitamin pill? However, NMC guidelines do permit a team discussion to be made regarding putting medication in food, in certain circumstances.

Staff argue that Mrs Hunter is keeping everybody else awake. Is this adequate justification for sedating her? A problem must be recorded in the care plan. If the home cannot cope it should not accommodate such residents. Then issues arise regarding reassessment for a placement elsewhere.

The Nurse Call System

Mrs Dainty repeatedly presses the nurse call button for what seem to be minor reasons such as moving an ornament. Indeed, she even presses the emergency buzzer! What can the nurse do?

To remove the buzzer would be some form of restraint, certainly if Mrs Dainty is unable to move herself. This would also be rather cruel and opposes the nurses' code of conduct as well as the public's expectations of the nurses' role. It may even be potentially harmful because the nurse would be unaware should Mrs Dainty need urgent assistance.

The nurse could attempt to explain the difficulties to Mrs Dainty and remind her that there are other residents. However, if Mrs Dainty uses the buzzer she is obviously in need of something. She may be bored or lonely for example. There may be an underlying source of anxiety of which the nurse is unaware. She may even be developing confusion and require medical assessment. The nurse may only discover the reason following discussions with Mrs Dainty and resulting action should be recorded. Records could also be kept of the times when Mrs Dainty uses the buzzer as perhaps there is some contributory factor; it may occur more frequently during ward reports, for example. Therefore a more satisfactory plan of care may be identified.

13 DECISIONS REGARDING PRESSURE CARE

Mr Griffith is in danger of developing pressure sores. The nurse insists upon standing him every one or two hours during the day since he is unable to move himself. However, Mr Griffith refuses to cooperate and insists that he will not be moved. What alternative action could be taken?

The nurse could discuss with Mr Griffith his reasons for this and the implications of not cooperating. Relatives could also be involved since they may be able to talk further with Mr Griffith. Perhaps Mr Griffith suffers pain when he is moved or does not like creating work for the nurses. Perhaps he feels that there is no purpose in life and thus no need to worry about pressure sores. Perhaps he wants to be the one in control. If he is in pain the nurse could obviously help to relieve it. Alternative methods of lifting may be of benefit. Perhaps he may wish to rest on his bed occasionally and additional pressure care aids could be utilised. The nurse could compromise with Mr Griffith, altering his position when he wants it and as he feels like it. Again it is essential to record action and outcomes within the nursing care plan which may be strengthened if the resident countersigned the notes. Indeed, the agreement of the plan of care by the resident or relative is a requirement of the Care Standards (2003). There have actually been court cases regarding the development of pressure sores due to failure to provide adequate nursing care (Waterlow, 1988).

Similarly Mrs Frost does not want to be woken two hourly throughout the night for pressure area care. Neither will a reduction in sleep contribute towards healing. Perhaps there is an alternative method of turning her with minimum disturbance, for example by using mechanical turning aids or the 30 degree tilt (Preston, 1988). An individual assessment must be undertaken; it may not be necessary to disturb her so frequently in the night at all.

Conversely Mrs Dean may request to have her position altered every 15 minutes. This should be discussed with Mrs Dean. She obviously has a need for something. Perhaps she is suffering from pain, boredom or loneliness. If the nurse does abide by Mrs Dean's request she may actually contribute towards the development of pressure sores. Ultimately, if it is not possible to compromise, Mrs Dean must be turned. Effectively she is refusing treatment that has been offered to her. The nurse must be able to indicate that all attempts have been made to provide prescribed nursing treatment; hence clear nursing notes must be made, again countersigned by Mrs Dean if possible. It would be of benefit to keep a record of the frequency of turns which may also serve as a reminder to Mrs Dean that she has indeed been turned.

14 DECISIONS REGARDING FIRE

Mrs Adaire desires to leave her bedroom door ajar. The nurse insists that she closes it, arguing that fire regulations insist upon it. Similarly, the lounge door is left open to permit independent movement of residents.

Fire officers may reconsider the requirement to keep all fire doors closed during certain situations such as regular use by residents; however, this must be discussed fully with all regulatory bodies. Indeed, there are automatic door closers which act when the fire alarm is activated. Closures can also be bought to hold doors open (Home Office Fire Department, 1983). As this department states, account must be taken of possible adverse effects of regulations on the quality of residents' lives and the care they receive (Home Office Fire Department, 1983). However, this guide does not possess legal stature. The closure of doors restricts residents' autonomy and independence and infringes their rights. Their doors would not be closed at home. However, there are many residents to consider within a home and the owners and staff fear litigation claims. It is dangerous to prop doors open with chairs or other objects. Until door closures are fitted if possible, the door must be kept closed in accordance with the Health and Safety Act (1974).

Mr Dent is to be admitted to the nursing home. He wishes to bring with him some personal items of furniture, for example his lamp, bed, table and chair. However, the home manager refuses to permit this, insisting that they are not fireproof and would clutter up the room, creating a fire hazard. It would also increase the difficulty of the domestic work.

The manager could have measured the room or offered to place the items in other areas of the home. This should be discussed with regulatory bodies, particularly fire officers, since if they are aware of the circumstances they may be flexible as discussed above. Policies do indeed differ per district.

Since Mr Dent has used that furniture for so long at home there should be no need to cease using it now. Abandoning it would create further distress for Mr Dent since the furniture may possess special meaning. It may also help to orientate him, promoting security and creating a more homely environment. Mr Dent may be accustomed to having a lot of furniture in his room. Surely it would be possible for the domestics to move the furniture and clean round it? Mr Dent may also be more likely to care for it himself, for example dusting, if permitted. Electrical items such as the lamp could be checked for safety before use. The majority of furniture is made of wood or wooden frames anyway, hence it is not totally fireproof. Indeed, every piece of furniture within a block of flats is not fireproof. However, foam-filled furniture is fire retardant since 1988. There is also fireproof spray.

It is fire practice and Mrs Swan, who is of sound mind, refuses to leave her room. The nurse is concerned about what would occur if this was a real fire.

If Mrs Swan is enforced physically this would be regarded as assault. If this was discussed with fire officers they may be prepared to make allowances for such residents and certainly for very ill residents, during fire practices. If a resident refused to leave the home during an actual fire, the firemen are legally able to remove the resident from the home anyway. The nurse must concentrate upon the safety of him or herself and other residents and staff.

Smoking

Mrs Roy requests a cigarette from a nurse but is told it is not cigarette time and she had one only an hour ago.

The nurse argues that if Mrs Roy alone is given one, everybody will want one; they will need observing due to fire risks and if they smoke too much they will suffer bad chests. Also smoke affects non-smoking individuals. Indeed, some residents have complained about residents who smoke. There are a number of issues here; fairness involving treating all residents alike, fire risk and prevention of ill health.

Whilst prevention is a national issue, what will be achieved by reducing the number of cigarettes smoked by a 70 or 80 year old? It is also more difficult to reduce the number smoked at that age, certainly when forced to do so. Indeed, on a wider scale some homes have banned smoking either by not admitting residents who smoke or requiring them to smoke outside which would make the resident even more susceptible to chest infections particularly if it is wet or cold weather. This also applies to staff.

Anybody may drop a cigarette causing fire but there are many individuals to consider within a nursing home. Whilst action must be undertaken to prevent fire it could be undertaken on a more individual scale. What alternative action could therefore be taken?

Mrs Roy could be permitted to keep her own cigarettes. Nurses are not in a position to legally withhold somebody's property which could again be regarded as theft. If the nurse withholds the matches only, somebody else may provide them. There is indeed an example of this occurring following which the patient burned to death within a hospital and the nurse was liable (Fiesta, 1988). A full assessment must be undertaken regarding Mrs Roy's actual needs – she may actually be fully capable of smoking alone. Smoking facilities must be available such as ashtrays and the area could be supervised frequently. It may be of benefit to discuss this with the fire officers, district health authorities and residents together to obtain understanding advice.

If Mrs Roy is provided with a cigarette but advised against smoking too many the nurse is fulfilling the prevention role but the outcome depends on Mrs Roy. Mrs Roy may not want to reduce her intake of cigarettes and the nurse must clarify his or her reasons for wishing her to do so.

To avoid disturbing non-smokers a designated smoking area could be utilised. However, this is reducing the autonomy of Mrs Roy since she desires to remain where she is but in doing so, she is reducing the autonomy of the majority. Such an area is also a form of segregation and may not assist those smokers who are attempting to reduce smoking. It should also not be a small uninspiring area.

Within some homes, residents are permitted to smoke

within their bedrooms. If the resident is safe there is no reason why not as long as it is not too near a smoke detector. Indeed, if residents were permitted to smoke with staff, for example in the lounge, it would be of immense social benefit creating opportunities to communicate as well as reducing staff-resident division.

Home owners do possess the right to refuse to admit certain residents, for example smokers. Indeed, ultimately they could give a resident notice of leave for disobeying such rules as 'no smoking'. Yet within a normal environment, there is a variety of individuals who smoke, drink or swear and where will it end? What about the married couple where one partner smokes and the other does not?

15 DECISIONS REGARDING RELATIONSHIPS

Mr and Mrs Hardy were a married couple who shared the same room. However, they were often heard to be arguing and the nurse was concerned particularly since Mrs Hardy had a few small but unexplained bruises.

The nurse cannot directly intervene. Indeed, arguments may worsen if the nurse does intervene. Little can be done to protect the elderly unless he or she asks for protection or is mentally incompetent.

The nurse must discuss this with Mrs Hardy; her assumption may be incorrect. She could suggest that assistance may be obtained but cannot obtain it without Mrs Hardy's consent. The police, however, may be able to initiate proceedings on behalf of a victim of abuse if too infirm or incapable of doing so him or herself (Griffiths *et al*, 1990). If a member of staff observes an attack he or she must intervene in order to protect Mrs Hardy. The problem must be recorded within the nursing care plan indicating that staff are aware and have acted as far as possible. An incident form must also be completed.

Similarly, two residents may be arguing. Whilst some individuals need to argue and it is also individual expression of emotion, the nurse may be able to suggest some form of compromise or diversion to prevent undue distress to both the residents concerned and remaining residents.

One resident makes sexual advances towards another. What could the nurse do?

There may be many situations like this and each must be considered on an individual basis involving the residents concerned.

If the resident dislikes the advances and in particular, objects to the behaviour, it may be considered as assault. In such a case the nurses must protect the resident by keeping them apart. However, it may be difficult if the resident is confused and fails to understand. He or she may even quite innocently mistake the other resident for their own husband or wife, now deceased.

Both residents may indeed be confused or potentially aggressive. The relationship may also be of a homosexual or lesbian nature, hence the nurse must not allow personal values and thoughts to colour ultimate action. For example, the home may have previously accommodated the partner and the staff feel very protective towards the resident. The majority of staff may be very young and the thought of such relationships may disgust them. It is, however, not for us or anybody else to judge (Dimon, 1999b).

Further, if the couple do wish to develop their relationship questions arise regarding the provision of a single room or privacy. They may even need assistance particularly if one or both of them are confined to wheelchairs.

Situations do arise where residents marry or wish to marry each other. Staff may find this difficult to accept regarding the above explanations. Relatives may also object but their motives may be questionable, for example reduction of their inheritance. Nor do relatives have any right to prevent such a marriage but the staff may not wish to upset relationships. Contact in this way, or even kissing, is a form of contact that reassures the sense of belonging. Indeed, what else would confused residents have? We are not suggesting that such relationships be actively encouraged but that they be accepted if they do occur. Ultimately the decision again belongs to the residents concerned. However, the situation must be discussed with staff to ensure that they understand and accept the situation. This is particularly important concerning the variety and amount of staff who work within homes.

Mr Wilson requests to have the company of a prostitute. What could the nurse do?

He has the right to do so in his own home but the nurse must consider the reputation of the home and the other residents. He could be allowed a discreet visit in his room or he may consider another place. There is actually a case of a home who arranged a prostitute for a resident (Nursing Times, 2004).

Decisions regarding relationships

Assisting Others

Mr Fox is buttoning Mrs Cole's cardigan up but is told not to
do so by the nurse. The nurse argues that Mrs Cole must do it
herself in order to maintain her independence. Surely there
are occasions when Mrs Cole will button it herself?

Whilst this will maintain Mrs Cole's physical independence
it will not promote her independence of mind or autonomy. Nor
does it assist Mr Fox's autonomy. Indeed, it may be compared
to extreme rehabilitation. This is physical rehabilitation, not
rehabilitation for living which involves the offer of help which
benefits both receiver and giver in order for it to be accepted.
By buttoning Mrs Cole's cardigan Mr Fox is fulfilling another
need, for that has priority over the mere buttoning of a
cardigan, such as the need for company.

Relatives

Mrs Green wishes to assist the nurse to lift her mother, Mrs
Jaques. The nurse refuses, informing Mrs Green of the risk of
back injury and the lack of insurance for Mrs Green, should
she herself be consequently injured. However, Mrs Green may
have cared for her mother for many months previously; even
if not she may still feel a need to assist. Indeed, her mother
may wish her to. Whilst the nurse is there to care primarily
for Mrs Jaques not Mrs Green, if Mrs Jaques wishes it then
she should permit it. Mrs Green could always be advised about
lifting and be supervised. Again the nursing records could be
countersigned by Mrs Green and her mother if necessary.
Similarly, she may wish to bath, wash or feed her mother. It
may be so much more comfortable for Mrs Jaques if so, since
she will be used to her daughter. However, all staff must be
aware of this in order to evaluate care, particularly if a problem
such as reluctance to eat exists. Hence, good communication
must be maintained between staff and relatives.

Noise

Mr Bird enjoys his radio but it disturbs the other residents. What action could be taken?

To remove the radio or batteries would be stealing. Another sitting room could be offered to Mr Bird or he could listen to the radio in his room. However, this would be restricting his autonomy since he desires to sit there. Times when the radio can be played may be restricted. Perhaps the volume could be turned down? Headphones for Mr Bird may be one solution. Indeed, could the remaining residents claim noise disturbance?

Reasons for the residents' annoyance must be discussed with them. If there is a residents' committee it may be a lively topic for discussion. Indeed, not all residents desire the same television channel or television to be turned on at all. Similarly, some homes have installed piped music which emits the noise of a radio station until a member of staff turns it off, but there are some systems with individual earphones.

Mrs Harris is an extremely confused and noisy lady. This disturbs the other residents. What could the nurse do?

It would be unfair and unethical to sedate her or even move her to another home for this reason. A full assessment must be undertaken to identify any pattern to this behaviour and hence possible cause or effective approach. The doctor and psychiatrist must be involved. Relatives, if there are any, could help to provide a past history to indicate possible reasons. A record must be made of the occurrences at onset and during Mrs Harris's behaviour and its duration as well as any possible allaying factors. Mrs Harris may at times like a change of scenery in her room, perhaps with a nurse sitting with her. However, it may not always be possible to sit with her. Peaceful music such as whale music could be played. Indeed, some homes possess a snoezelen room for this purpose (Hope, 2004). Adopting a person-centred care approach (Kitwood and Bredin in Bruce et al, 2002) would involve a holistic approach and listening to Mrs Harris. The challenge within a care home is considering the many individuals who live there.

16 DECISIONS REGARDING PERSONAL CARE

Mrs Graves refuses to have her weekly bath yet again. The nurse insists upon it arguing that she has not had a bath for a month and if she begins to smell it will be distressing for the other residents. Indeed, she may even be covered in faeces.

To force Mrs Graves into a bath is assault and it may particularly occur regarding confused residents thus worsening their confusion. It is similar to enforcing treatment; however, this is nurse treatment not medical treatment. What alternative action could have been taken?

Whilst gentle persuasion may have succeeded, the incident may recur in the future and it may not solve the problem from Mrs Graves' perspective.

There may be various reasons for refusing a bath and it is essential to explore all possibilities. It may signify depression or even embarrassment. Are male carers present? Would she prefer her own relatives to assist her? It is essential to be aware of the resident's past history. She may never have had a bath at home for example. She may be frightened of the bath itself, never having seen a bath with a hoist. Perhaps she would prefer to have a shower? An all-over wash is just as beneficial.

Ultimately if a bath is still refused even if urgently required, that is Mrs Graves' decision but action taken must be recorded thus protecting the nurse. A bath can always be offered at a different time of day; perhaps she would prefer one just before going to bed?

Conversely Mr Savage requests an additional bath. This is not permitted because he has already had one and there is a lack of time. Surely there is time somewhere and Mr Savage does enjoy a bath.

Mrs Skin requests to bath alone without the presence of care staff. However, the nurse insists upon being present because she may fall down or become scalded, for example. What alternative action could have been taken?

The nurse could regularly check Mrs Skin. However, this is still reducing her privacy and is in opposition to Mrs Skin's desires.

Reasons for wishing to bath alone should be explored. Perhaps the resident is embarrassed by the presence of a member of the opposite sex. Perhaps she merely prefers to bath alone, this being what she is used to.

If the reasons for wishing to remain with Mrs Skin are discussed with her and full records made within the nursing care plan, the nurse will be protected. A risk assessment must also be done. If able, Mrs Skin could sign an agreement but this may not be absolute protection for the nurse.

The bathroom must be adequately prepared beforehand such as nurse-call buzzer nearby and Mrs Skin could perhaps call for a nurse if she requires assistance when getting out of the bath.

Water from the taps should never be scalding hot. The recommended temperature (Health and Safety Executive, 1993) is 43 degrees C and mixer taps are suggested, commencing with cold water. Warning signs may also be displayed. Indeed, a hospital was found to be liable when a patient was scalded because the water was too hot within the system (Fiesta, 1988) although this was in the USA where the legal system may be different from that in Britain.

Similarly Mr Sprat desires to bath alone but requires the bath hoist to put him into the bath. There is no reason why he could not be left with the nurse-call buzzer nearby to use when he is ready to get out. This may be supported by a full individual assessment including an assessment of the risks involved, again recommended by the Health and Safety Executive (1993).

There may be cases when a resident, suffering from epilepsy for example, wishes to bath alone. A full assessment of the risks involved incorporating the resident's views and desires must be undertaken. Ultimately treatment cannot be enforced but there may be compromises such as knocking upon the bathroom door at intervals or waiting outside.

Decisions regarding personal care

Residents are not permitted to possess their own razors because they may cut themselves.

Again individual assessments must be undertaken. The resident could be supervised if necessary and if in agreement.

Most people like to shave themselves particularly since they have done so for most of their lives. Indeed, the nurse may cut the resident and if razors are kept by staff, there is a danger of cross infection.

Mrs Bean refuses to change her clothes; they may even be stained with the remains of an earlier meal. Perhaps she is anxious about the amount of laundry or clothes being mislaid. The resident may also be embarrassed about somebody else washing their dirty linen. Indeed, some residents hide their dirty clothes or wash their own underwear for this reason. Reassurance could be provided here, possibly introducing the resident to the laundry staff. He or she may be able to wash some of their clothes themselves but that is another issue. An incentive to change her clothes such as trips out would also help. The resident may not possess many clothes that he or she enjoys wearing or they may not fit.

Maintaining a resident's quality of life may thus conflict with the quality of care expected to be provided by the nurse. The nurse for example may fear reprimands from the following shift, from matron or from the relatives if the resident is seen in a dirty clothes. Indeed, the nursing home inspector may be due to visit.

Is a good home one in which all residents wear clean clothes similar to a uniform or one in which residents are prepared to be individuals?

Mr Haigh refuses to remove his dentures when going to bed. What could the nurse do?

The nurse may argue that they ought to be removed because he may choke on them during the night or they will impede any necessary resuscitation attempts.

The nurse may advise the resident. To forcibly remove the dentures would be assault.

The reasons for the resident's refusal should be explored; he may fear losing them or may never have removed them at home for example. However, the resident is not obliged to provide a reason. Ultimately the dentures must be left in. All action must be recorded within the nursing care plan indicating that the nurse is aware and has attempted to do something.

Mr Dark refuses to allow the nurse to cut his nails, which are rather long. What could the nurse do?

1. Enforce him;
2. Ask another nurse to hold his hands down;
3. Cut them when he is asleep.

To enforce Mr Dark would be abuse. Mr Dark has made a decision and his rights must be maintained. However, the nurse must try to encourage him to have them cut. If the resident is confused, at present the legal situation remains the same. It is unclear yet whether or not the Mental Capacity Act will refer to such decisions. However, an approach is being considered by the Government termed 'protective care' (Age Concern Bulletin, 2005).

A problem must be documented in the care plan, stating that he will not have his nails cut and records made of what was done about it. The nurse must consider alternatives. Possibly he would prefer somebody else, or a relative, to cut them? It may be better to cut them after a bath when they are softer. Perhaps he would like a change of environment or a peaceful atmosphere? If the problem is his toe nails, he may permit the chiropodist to cut them. Most chiropodists will not cut finger nails.

The Hoist

Mr Drummond will not permit the nurse to lift him using the hoist since he dislikes it. What could the nurse do?

This is a difficult situation. An employee is under duty to maintain his or her own safety and that of others and two nurses must not transfer the weight of anyone above 50kg (RCN, 2002). The employer also has responsibilities according to the health and safety regulations (1993). Effectively the nurse could refuse to transfer the resident and the employer could not enforce the nurse to do so. Indeed, the home manager could actually refuse to care for Mr Drummond, thus requiring him to seek care elsewhere. However, Mr Drummond also has rights. It would be assault if the nurse put Mr Drummond in the hoist against his wishes.

There may be various reasons why he will not permit the nurse to use the hoist. Perhaps he feels undignified and lacks privacy. If so there are alternative ways of covering him up. The sling may not be the correct size or type. There are various types of slings and hoists and they may be used on a trial basis. The staff's lifting technique should be reassessed. Again, this must be recorded in the care plan as a problem. A risk assessment must also be done (RCN, 2003).

17 DECISIONS REGARDING BEDTIME

Mr Dove is very tired and requests to go to bed at 6 pm. The nurse refuses explaining that it is too early and he will not sleep at night. What alternative action could be taken?

The nurse could explore why he wants to go to bed early; he could be bored, have been up since 6am or be feeling unwell. Perhaps he would like an afternoon nap in future? A full assessment of Mr Dove's sleep pattern is essential. What was his normal sleep pattern at home and what is it now?

The nurse must be aware of the foundations for her response. Perhaps he or she objects to being seemingly told what to do by a resident. Mr Dove may be an unpopular resident or is it a busy time? It is possible that night staff are complaining because residents are awake at night. Some matrons have banned going bed before 7pm for example or will not permit afternoon naps for this reason. However, sleep patterns alter with aging; the duration of sleep is reduced because less sleep is necessary, the main requirement being for growth and repair. Hence short naps are common (Wilson, 2003). Matron must also examine his or her reasons. Does he or she assume that staff want to put residents to bed early for their own benefit so they can have a crafty cup of tea for example?

Similarly, Mrs Dear wants a lie in bed but is told to get up because she will miss breakfast and the room wants cleaning. We all like lie in at some time, certainly if there appears to be little to get up for; imagine not having a job to go to, for example.

Couldn't breakfast be kept for her? Would she like toast in bed? This is another issue – why not?

Again her normal getting up time must be noted; there should be no reason to alter this. The room could be cleaned later or on another day. Mrs Dear may even like to clean it herself and that is another issue.

Mr Grant refuses to get up at all. What forms of action are available?

Again it is unacceptable to physically force him out of bed. This would be assault (Dimon, 1999a). It would be far better to explore reasons which may include boredom, depression or the need for peace for example. The nurse must still regularly check Mr Grant if he does remain in bed, taking him his meals and drinks and not avoid him, hoping that he will get up realising that he is achieving nothing. This should not be a battle between nurse and resident. If Mr Grant has a need we are there to help him fulfil it.

Similarly a resident may get up at 4am. Perhaps he has regularly got up at this time, certainly if his job was a milkman or farmer for example.

Some homes do not permit residents to go to their room during the day. It is argued that this contributes towards rehabilitation and residents may never leave their room otherwise.

Such rehabilitation attempts may actually cause regression by removing the residents' desire to be rehabilitated. Some residents may prefer their own company and do not always desire to be amongst others.

The nurse concentrates upon physical rehabilitation at expense of psychological rehabilitation. If it opposes the autonomy of the resident it is pointless. It is also a form of restraint or confinement.

Hot Water Bottles

Mr Jones would like a hot water bottle in his bed. However, the nurse will not permit him to use one. It is argued that he may be scalded by the bottle or it may burst. Mr Jones may be accustomed to using a hot water bottle, having used one regularly at home. It may provide him with additional comfort or he may indeed be cold.

Whatever the reason, Mr Jones wishes to use a hot water bottle.

Scalds may be prevented by not overfilling the bottle, using water of an appropriate temperature and not using an old bottle. All action taken must be recorded within the nursing care plan and a risk assessment completed. Advice given must be recorded with Mr Jones's, response and ultimate action. Again this could be countersigned by Mr Jones but this should be unnecessary.

There have been two such cases in the USA that the author is aware of: a hot water bottle scalded a patient because it was too hot (1948) and one was improperly capped (1949) (Fiesta, 1988) thus substantiating the nurse's fears.

18 DECISIONS REGARDING INCONTINENCE

During the night all residents are woken every two hours to put them on the toilet. This is said to prevent incontinence. It does not prevent incontinence. It merely prevents a wet bed thus reducing wet linen and nurses' inconvenience. This is invasion of residents' privacy and in opposition of their right to sleep. Indeed, they may take civil action against the nurse, including assault, particularly if they have expressed a desire not to be woken.

Alternatively individual assessments could be undertaken. Are certain residents always incontinent at night and if so how often? If the individual frequency of micturition was noted the resident could at least be changed as soon as possible.

Mr Crawford requests to go to the toilet during the day but is told that he cannot do so because he has recently been and it is not toilet time yet.

A full assessment must again be undertaken. Possibly Mr Crawford has an infection or is a diabetic? It may be an excuse for a walk or something to do. He may be seeking reassurance that the nurse is there for him. The nurse must be aware of his usual pattern of micturition, preferably on admission. Whatever the reason, Mr Crawford wishes to go to the toilet now, even if during mealtimes. Not to attend to him is a form of professional negligence since the nurse is not fulfilling his or her role as expected.

Mrs Evans is frequently wet through due to urinary incontinence. However, matron refuses to permit her to wear pads against staff requests, even though Mrs Evans previously wore pads at home. There are no pads within the nursing home. Matron assumes that if residents wore pads, staff would not change them. This also applies to draw sheets upon the beds. What can staff do?

Mrs Evans' incontinence must be assessed for frequency and possible treatment involving the area incontinence advisor if there is one. Certainly reasons for incontinence must be explored, and it may be due to medication (Nazarko, 1995). Who would pay for such pads must be considered since the home owner does not always provide them. Ultimately if Mrs Evans does require pads it is the home's responsibility to ensure that care is provided as required and it may be necessary to involve the care home inspector. Some matrons insist that urinary catheters be inserted for this reason. This would be regarded as assault, certainly if it opposed Mrs Evans' wishes or recommendations of the incontinence advisor. Urinary catheters should be a last resort since they are a potential source of infection, reduce dignity and are likely to be long term if inserted for this purpose. Whilst there are alternatives staff should inform the GP of such use of catheters since they will be provided out of his or her budget.

Now incontinence pads are provided by the NHS based upon assessment by an incontinence nurse. However, issues arise regarding this. In some districts, pads are not provided for faecal incontinence. Nor are pads provided for use at night. Yet items such as draw sheets are inappropriate for some residents. Again, decisions need to be made on an individual basis. The home manager must keep individual records and approach the Primary Care Trust.

19 OTHER DECISIONS

Decisions Regarding Pets

Mrs Hunt is not permitted to bring her pet dog into the home. Staff argue that it is unhygienic, it will need attending to and other residents will not like it. Many homes do not permit pets and there are cases of residents remaining at home because of this (Nursing Times, 1994).

There are advantages to having pets such as reduction of boredom, confusion, depression and loneliness, and encouragement of exercise (Walster, 1982). Whilst it could be argued that it is unhygienic a home ought not to be an overtly clinical environment and it could be kept away from kitchens and treatment rooms. Perhaps an enclosed area could be provided for it outside. If it was a cat it would self care to some degree and volunteers may also be involved. Not all residents would dislike it but nothing can be assumed until the animal arrives. If there is a residents committee this could be a subject for discussion. Some individuals may however be allergic to animals. Budgerigars seem to be more commonly accepted, possibly because they require less attention and are not free to roam. Ultimately if the home manager will not accept the pet, the resident must consider another home provided there is one in that locality. There is a trust which will provide a list of residential homes which do accept pets.

Decisions Regarding Locks

Very few nursing home managers permitted residents to lock their bedroom door (Counsel and Care, 1991). Homes are now required to fit them according to the Care Standards (2003). Reasons for not providing them include: there are no locks, the resident would lose his or her key or would collapse when the door is locked. This also applies to the toilet doors. This creates a lack of privacy, dignity, choice and respect as a person. Indeed, other people may wander into the room including visitors and other residents.

If there are no locks they could easily be obtained and there is a variety to select from, for example there are locks that may be opened from the outside during an emergency. There are also locks which the physically disabled are able to use. Nursing staff could also possess a master key. Latches and chains may also be used; indeed, it will be possible to force them open during an emergency.

The fact that personal keys for residents are more commonly permitted in residential homes than in nursing homes may indicate that this decision may be dependent upon the physical ability of the residents, since those within residential homes are theoretically more independent than those within nursing homes.

However, this is not supported by the common misplacement of residents into either type of home. It is therefore essential to base such decisions upon individual assessments of residents.

A resident always kept a chair behind the bedroom door at home. Whilst the nurse was initially concerned, following discussion with the remainder of the team and the resident this was able to be continued. It was, however, recorded within the care plan and a risk assessment done.

Decisions Regarding Pocket Money

Few residents within nursing or residential homes are permitted to possess their own money (Counsel and Care, 1992). It is now a requirement, according to the Care Standards (2003), that they do have money. Whilst the nurse has limited control of this issue directly, he or she is required by the Nursing and Midwifery Council (NMC), if a qualified nurse, to request personal allowances for the resident from the home owner or the resident's relative. All residents should have a personal weekly allowance according to the National Assistance Act 1948.

A resident who goes out may not have any money. Some nurses argue that residents would lose it, or not know what to spend it on. Apart from loss of independence, not to have money in their pocket is the equivalent of vagrancy to some. This will therefore involve a great loss of pride and dignity.

Some home managers argue that the home provides everything such as soap and hairdressing. The residents and relatives may not be aware of this and the resident should certainly be given the choice of which hairdresser to use. It is preferable that the resident goes out and chooses what to buy. However, not all homes do provide toiletries. That is another issue.

Nursing staff should speak to the resident and identify what he or she desires. Residents could be provided with locked drawers for money and other valuables; however, this very rarely occurs (Counsel and Care 1992). It is now required according to the Care Standards (2003) but not all residents want a locked drawer.

Neither residents nor relatives may be aware of regulations regarding personal allowances, but Age Concern do offer an advisory line and further information.

There are occasions when a resident's relative will not release the money. Indeed, they or the owners may be saving for the resident's funeral. In this case it may be necessary to involve a social worker.

It is possible to safeguard the financial interests of residents. Regarding mentally disordered individuals, the Court of Protection appoints a receiver who is usually a relative or friend. It is not recommended that anybody connected with running the home be appointed as a receiver. (Age Concern, 1986). If the resident is mentally ill, a guardian may be appointed. Alternatively, if the resident is capable of understanding, a Power of Attorney may be appointed to care for his or her finances. An Enduring Power of Attorney may be appointed should the resident become incompetent (Age Concern, 1986).

Money may be collected by an agent who is usually the home owner or resident's relative. However, this most commonly occurs because the resident is unaware of alternatives; certainly if he or she does not have any relatives.

If the resident is affected by this, for example is unable to buy anything due to not having any money, this is a problem for that resident and should be recorded as such within the care plan. Hence a plan of action must be identified and evaluated.

Decisions Regarding Sewing

Mrs Byrne would like to sew with her sewing machine. What could the nurse do?

A risk assessment is essential. There are risks to Mrs Byrne who may sew her finger. There may also be risks to other residents. The nurse could ensure that there is a lock on Mrs Byrne's door, to prevent other residents from touching the sewing machine, or harming themselves on it, and consider what supervision is available. Mrs Byrne could sign a disclaimer but again the legality of this is questionable. Ultimately Mrs Byrne has a right to use her sewing machine and the benefits for her may outweigh any actual risk.

20 DISCUSSION

There are issues that exist nationally and are affected by socio-political factors. There is evidence of their historical existence, for example home size. If there were no issues, development would cease because nothing would be questionable and hence alternatives not considered.

Decisions and dilemmas in care homes are not helped by various factors. The fundamental issue is the role of long-term care and the nurse. There are few definitions of long-term care, hence the specific role of the nurse within this area remains obscure.

Present definitions include:

The provision of services – physical, psychological, spiritual, environmental and economic – needed to help people attain, maintain or retain their optimum level of functioning (Abdellah in Copp, 1981).

Any premises used or intended to be used for the reception of and provision of nursing for persons suffering from any sickness, injury, infirmity (Registered Homes Act, 1984) and now the Care Standards Act (2000).

One or more services provided on a sustained basis to enable individuals whose functional capacities are chronically impaired to be maintained at their maximum levels of health and wellbeing (Brody, 1977).

An institution providing a protective and supervised environment, licensed to care (American College of Nursing Home Administration in Schmidt Kayser-Jones, 1981).

Generally, these definitions are of two types defining either the actual structure (Registered Homes Act, 1984) or the aim of long-term care (Abdellah in Copp, 1981). If we define what the service actually is there is a danger of defining the service before identifying the actual needs of the residents. Defining what the service ought to be does provide an actual aim, direction and motivation to promote development. However, who defines aim?

According to Abdellah in Copp, 1981, the aim is optimum level of functioning. Whilst service providers must consider the majority, surely individuals can be considered at local level. For the author, therefore, long-term care refers to the provision of holistic care within a homely environment in order to maintain the individual resident's quality of life which is equated with autonomy.

The role of long-term care must be determined by the need for it and not vice versa, in order to be of any value and to prevent exclusion of certain individuals or adjustment of individuals to fit defined aims, categories or needs. Indeed, this is the focal issue of the NHS and Community Care Act (1990), to provide a service in response to needs. Whereabouts to care for older people at all is the issue; presently the aim is within their own homes. These aims do have cost implications. However, community care is not necessarily cheaper (Kirkevoid and Engedal, 2005) although this depends upon what community care consists of. Despite the fact that only six per cent of elderly reside within long-term care establishments (Shukla, 1999), care homes will always be necessary due to inadequate community care for example, in addition to the increasing number of elderly and family dispersal. Therefore they must not be forgotten. Apart from that, nursing homes exist now and the issues within them must not be ignored. Even the quality of only one person's life is of value.

In all cases nurses have provided a rationale when asked. However, this is based upon their viewpoint only at that time. Whilst nurses think that they are doing the right thing, there are alternative courses of action that may be suggested by other nurses or staff, the resident or the relatives of the resident. In all cases it is essential to speak to or consider the resident or if this is not possible, the resident's advocate. If the well-meaning nurse opposes the resident's wishes, it becomes unintentional abuse.

Discussion

Common rationales for the actions refer to fairness to all residents, ease of the nurse and reluctance of the nurse to take risks. It is therefore vital that all action taken, including discussions with the resident, is recorded within the care plan. Recording the rationale for that action will ensure that all staff are aware of the reasons as well as indicating that it has been professionally considered. It may also indicate whether or not additional thought is required. If a rationale cannot be stated for that action preferably incorporating a resident's or advocate's opinion, then it must not be taken unless in an emergency situation. The fact that the issues were inappropriately resolved indicates that individual assessments were lacking or inappropriately undertaken. Re-assessments are also important as residents' needs and wishes may change. Indeed, one of the most common law suits concerns failure to assess the patient and to record adequate history (Douglass, 1992). It is essential to record the resident's past history and present goals or desires which may influence his or her decision-making and enable the nurse to empathise to a greater degree. The nurse must be aware of any personal opinions which may bias suggested action. Discussing the outcome with a second nurse may assist this. Indeed, the wishes of certain individuals may be opposed, for example an additional cup of tea because of his or her unpopularity with the nurse (Finlay, 2005). This may particularly be so within long-term care because residents may be more dependant than within acute areas, may be confused and the nurses care for the same residents for a greater length of time. Since the residents are also in a relatively unchanging nursing home situation, they may appear to be more demanding in certain ways because they require additional psychological support, depending upon how or indeed if they have adjusted individually. Also one individual is not aware of all possible solutions. There are various courses of action and it is necessary to consider as many as possible before acting. Nurses need to be creative and flexible.

Whilst care plans are so important they are underused and often not written in at all (Shea, 1986). More specifically, records are often not made regarding the decision to conceal medication in food (Kirkevoid and Engedal, 2005). Staff in these cases are exposed to possible lawsuits.

There are many reasons given for nurses failing to write in care plans, such as lack of time, ignorance or fear of being held accountable (De La Cuesta, 1983). Therefore nurses need support from their colleagues and manager. The registered manager, who is ultimately responsible, needs to undertake care plan audits to identify that records have been made (Appendix 2).

The most common rationale was reluctance to take risks, or nurses' fear of reprimands if anything untoward did occur as indicated by the reference to regulations and nurses' inflexibility. Therefore a risk assessment must be completed for the individual resident such as Mr Soames who wishes to bathe alone (Appendix 3). This entails considering the environment, equipment and education necessary in order to indicate to the nurse or Mr Soames any possible risks and solutions. If all staff together completed a risk assessment for themselves, this would indicate what the fundamental reason was for failing to adhere to the resident's wishes, which may in reality be unjustified.

Other possible reasons for nurses failing to promote residents' autonomy include adherence to the medical model (Wade et al, 1983). This concerns such issues as enforced reducing diets and is unaided by society's emphasis upon stopping smoking, losing weight and healthy diets (Department of Health, 1998). Routine provision of care is still evident within establishments (Wade et al, 1983). Whilst routine may reduce nurse anxiety (Menzies, 1970) it may increase anxiety for others. Some nurses can avoid decision making by adhering to routine.

Indeed, children have been permitted more freedom than the elderly as indicated by reference to the Children's Act such as self medication. This is possibly affected by their perceived roles in society, for example children are developing; however, people possess equal rights as human beings. Increasing the freedom of the elderly residents may also reduce the physical amount of work required of the nurse as well as increasing the motivation of both staff and residents for example. Patient decision making is now promoted but in an NHS orientated publication (Department of Health, 2001). Similarly person-centred care involves listening to patients (Department of Health, 2005). Such guidelines need to refer to care homes.

A conflict between the rights and safety of residents is indicated. However, it is the right of the individual resident not to maintain personal safety in this way. Therefore it may actually be conflicting with the rights, safety and expectations of the nurse.

The rationale for action must be isolated from the personal aims or needs of the nurse. For example, the nurse may desire to control other individuals or situations.

The issues exist because the resident has refused nursing treatment as opposed to medical treatment, for example Mrs Blue's failure to walk. Whilst this supports the claim for unique nursing knowledge certainly within long-term care, it identifies the absolute necessity to include the resident in that decision. Residents must not be excluded from the formation of a nursing diagnosis since this would be an identifying problem to the nurse, not the resident.

Primary nursing may assist individual decision making (Armitage et al, 1999) since the primary nurse is primarily responsible for a smaller number of residents, usually four, hence possessing more knowledge regarding them personally. This is not possible within the majority of nursing homes due to the low number of qualified nurses. The key worker system is an alternative, involving resident to carer to nurse allocation. However, one nurse still has the decision to make at the time if aware; occasionally the care assistant decides unknown to the nurse. The possibility of this may be increased by the care assistant's sense of responsibility for those certain residents. Therefore it must be carefully applied and evaluated. Hence the effect of this depends upon the individual nurse and support from colleagues to a large degree.

Noticeably the inspectors themselves are excluded from the resolving of such issues by the nurse. This is an indication of the need for inspectors to be available informally, at local level in order to advise and support nurses who should also be prepared and unafraid to consult them.

Whilst nurses do consider that their action is taken to protect the residents it is not always effective because residents' perceptions differ and there are many factors to consider. Maintenance of residents' physical safety may conflict with promotion of autonomy but what is the purpose of maintaining safety without autonomy? Without autonomy quality of life is negligible since the individual has no choice of the direction or form of his or her life. An obvious conflict between nurses' and residents' aims exists, primarily quantity or quality of life. In failing to take risks the nurse is opposing residents' autonomy and is therefore in danger of being confronted by legal action. Whilst the majority of residents are not in a position physically, psychologically or financially to do this, the possibility of this may increase with the advance of advocacy and public awareness. However, nurses also have the majority of residents to consider as will be further discussed. Nurses must also consider residents' relatives and indeed members of the public; for example, what would their reaction be if Mr Day was knocked down by a car and killed? Nurses are ultimately responsible for the residents but re-education of the public and discussion with relatives are necessary. Therefore there are many reasons for actions taken

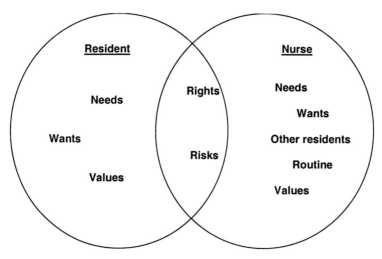

Figure 1

Discussion

by the nurse, essentially: personal values, social values, organisational values, personal needs and needs of other residents – thus determining the rights and risks that are taken. Nurses must be aware of the fundamental reason in order to achieve an effective outcome. Whilst education determines the awareness of alternatives the actual selection depends upon the above factors. Comparatively the resident has only him or herself to consider (Fig 1).

21 CONCLUSION

Many issues within nursing homes remain unaddressed by professionals and politicians hence confusion continues to exist. As indicated, some issues may be regarded as abuse if ineffectively resolved, for example restraint (HMSO, 1992). However, there are situations in which some form of restraint may be necessary thus indicating further the necessity to think before acting. Blanket application of rules, such as prohibiting smoking or eating within residents' own rooms, should cease since this does not address individual needs at all.

All types of issues exist because there are various possible solutions and various rationales that may be provided. Hence there is a danger of creating issues unnecessarily. Should some situations actually be issues at all? For example, why shouldn't Mrs Skin bath alone? This highlights the importance of identifying the fundamental aim of care. Are we aiming to promote health or safety or autonomy?

The number of issues increases as knowledge increases because there are many possible solutions and hence more alternatives to select from. The source of issues increases with the increasing number of older people and nursing homes. The nurse may aim for quantity of life considering only the needs of residents, from the nurse's perspective. Since the resident does not want to adhere to a diet for example, aiming for quality of life is not a personal need for him or her. Therefore there is a difference between needs and wants. The outcome of all needs is wanted but not all wants are needed.

Each nurse's decision depends upon various factors as discussed; even more so if specific guidelines do not exist. Ultimately the nurse alone makes the decision to permit or to prohibit. To provide some form of direction, some homes possess a philosophy of care. It is now a requirement (Care Standards, 2003) for care homes to have a service-user guide

81

incorporating this. Homes must also have policies of care. The benefit of this depends upon the method of its application and formation which should include all staff and residents and their advocates thus considering the opinions of various people. It should also be reviewed regularly to promote usage and understanding. Whilst similar issues do exist between homes it would be beneficial to communicate and exchange ideas. The existence of a nursing home development group would contribute enormously to this (Salvage, 1989). Nurses within nursing homes are particularly isolated by competition of home owners or managers, position or low number of qualified nurses for example. The competitive nature of some nursing home managers must reduce. Some home managers, for example, cling onto their ideas to prevent other homes from offering the same but this may work both ways. Indeed, home managers could be required to indicate how they have contributed towards long-term care knowledge in this way. Education is essential regarding the decision-making process including the involvement of residents as well as the subject in question (Reece and Walker, 2000). Methods of education include reflection and role-play which may promote self-awareness of nurses, particularly regarding moral behaviour. Education should not provide a prescription of actions since all situations differ. A good nurse is one who considers all possible alternatives recognising that no one person possesses all the correct answers. It is this process that education must promote. Life itself is about decisions and decision making. Therefore this decision-making process must be learned. Is long-term care unpopular because nurses are unable to identify instant solutions to problems and need to feel that they are achieving something as occurs more frequently within acute care? Whilst there is no nationally accepted definition of long-term care, decisions will be difficult to make because their aim is unclear. The definition must be applicable and acceptable though and not, for example, to cure. Nurses and policy makers must recognise who they exist for and act accordingly. It is essential to include resi-dents in all decisions affecting their care as is evident throughout this book. If residents are incapable, their advocates may be included, for example a nurse, relative or advocacy group.

Actions may depend upon regulations but to what extent is this really so? For example, nurses may not permit residents to smoke within their bedrooms although the regulations of each district vary and fire officers may adopt an understanding and flexible approach. Nurses must approach regulatory bodies more for advice and they must be approachable and supportive, otherwise an additional, intermediary body is required. Since these are individual situations the nurse needs independence, knowledge and support in order to respond. Clinical nurse specialists or consultant nurses may also offer advice and support. However, whilst there are some specifically for care homes, there need to be more (Harrison, 2004).

Nursing homes are required by an increasing number of older people and because of their vulnerability and potential issues, ultimate responsibility must be adopted by a general body. Even though the majority of homes are not publicly owned, the government is still responsible to ensure that services are available for the individuals who require them. Hence they must provide direction by definite policies and action. There is evidence that this is not occurring. Since some of these issues have historically existed, there is a need for action to be taken. Whilst flexibility is required, as illustrated by smoking regulations for example, inspectors and people working within care homes require more definite direction.

There is a need for a human rights commission to protect and promote human rights. Indeed, there is little awareness of human rights in care homes (Watson, 2002). A charter of residents' rights would be beneficial (Dimon, 2002) as exists in America.

Ultimately, if issues are resolved unsatisfactorily, the resident and advocate must be aware of the complaints procedure. Nurses must also be aware of how they may complain, possibly on behalf of the resident. It is a requirement of the Care Standards (2003) to have a clear complaints procedure. If approaching the manager or owner achieves nothing the care home inspector or NMC may be informed. Whilst all individuals must be supported should this occur,

Conclusion

whether he or she does complain or not is another issue. Nurses cannot and must not ignore these issues since they affect the care provided. Their occurrence further highlights the necessity for the nurse to reject adopted models of medicine or administration and identify their own unique role within long-term care primarily to practise in partnership with those with whom he or she cares, identifying needs and action with the resident. This has major implications for the remainder of nursing; if the nurse cannot identify a role within this area there is little hope for the role of nursing and indeed caring.

It should not just be the fear of civil action that prevents the nurse from undertaking the correct action. All nurses must examine their values and views and be prepared to be flexible in response to the individual situation. Whilst there may be additional factors to consider, surely some agreement can be reached? For example, if Mrs Snow requests caviar it can obviously not be provided regularly but perhaps it may be given upon special occasions or be paid for out of home funds or Mrs Snow's allowance with her agreement. If we cannot assist residents to achieve personal aims, what are we there for? Possibly an approach similar to the hospice concept could be adopted (Kayser-Jones *et al*, 2005) but it may promote an image of dependency.

These situations indicate the number and variety of decisions nurses and care assistants make and are involved in. Therefore care in care homes is highly skilled. Nurses and care assistants require skills of decision making as well as of the aspects of care concerned. A skilled individual is able to consider alternatives and identify possible outcomes (Baron, 1988) (Figure 2). However, it must also be a team decision.

Nurses must accept and confront the challenges of these issues but to do so they require support from each other, allied professionals, hierarchy, residents and their advocates and the public. Behind every nursing action there is a decision the aim of which is to nurse but what does 'to nurse' mean or indeed, 'to care'? That is the ultimate question for which an answer is urgently required.

There may be many more issues that you are aware of. Hopefully this book will assist the decision-making process. If

Decisions and Dilemmas in Care Homes

you are able to identify additional issues within your own area, then something has been achieved.

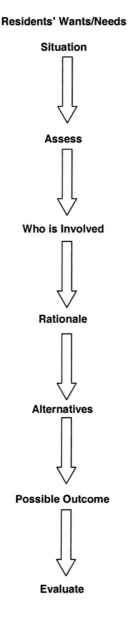

Residents' Wants/Needs

Situation

Assess

Who is Involved

Rationale

Alternatives

Possible Outcome

Evaluate

Figure 2

22 RECOMMENDATIONS

In summary, the following recommendations may be made:

1. Education for qualified and training nurses and unqualified staff, involving role-play, reflection and such methods that may promote self-awareness and self-control. Education regarding the decision-making process and promotion of flexibility.

2. Support from nurses, hierarchy, allied professionals, members of the public, residents and their advocates.

3. Regulatory bodies to advise, assist and support as well as to regulate.

4. Awareness of district and other district policies in order to present the facts to owners, managers or inspectors.

5. Definition and philosophy of long-term care and the role of the nurse to direct actions and decisions.

6. Nursing home philosophies must involve all staff and residents and their advocates and must be used and reviewed, not hidden.

7. Meetings to promote discussion and exploration of decisions. This would identify alternatives as well as reduce fear.

8. Quality assurance if it includes all staff, residents and their advocates, and addresses such issues.

9. Awareness of complaints procedure by staff and residents.

10. Care plans record actions, rationale and outcome as well as evaluations. They must be very clearly written. A section for residents' perceptions or comments could be included.

These should be countersigned by resident or advocate if necessary.

11. Risk assessments must be done and reviewed regularly.

12. Consultation of other nursing staff, additional professionals and regulatory bodies when making certain decisions.

13. A charter of rights for residents in care homes.

23 REFERENCES

Age Concern (1986)
The Law and Vulnerable Elderly People
Age Concern Bulletin (May 2005)
'Commission for social care inspection and healthcare commission to be merged' p46
Age Concern Bulletin (May 2005)
'Mental Capacity Act' p8
Age Concern Bulletin (May 2005)
'Bournewood case: Approach to be taken' p44
Age Concern Bulletin (Oct 2004)
Assessment of care needs and the Human Rights Act' p27
Agich GJC (1993)
Autonomy in long-term care
Oxford University Press
Armitage P, Champney-Smith J, Andrews K (1991)
Journal of Advanced Nursing v16 pp413–422
'Primary nursing and the role of the nurse preceptor in changing longterm mental healthcare, an evaluation'
Baron J (1988)
Thinking and deciding
Cambridge University Press
Bennett G, Kingston P (1993)
'Elder Abuse: Concepts, Theories and Interventions'
Chapman and Hall, Canada
Bolling Maynard B, Woehle RE, Heilman JE (1977)
Better homes for the aged
Lexington Books
Booth T (1985)
Home Truths: Old People's Homes and Outcomes of Care
Gower, Hants
Brazier M (1992)
Medicines, patients and the law
Penguin Books, London

Brody EM (1977)
Long-term Care of Older People
Human Sciences Press, USA

Bruce E, Surr C, Tibbs M, Downs M (2002)
Nursing Times Research v7 n5 pp335–347
Bradford Dementia Group
'Moving towards a special kind of care for people with dementia living in care homes'

Burger JM (1989)
Journal of personal and social psychology v56 n2 pp246–256
'Negative reactions to increases in perceived control'

Butterworth C (2005)
Nursing Standard Jan 26 v 19 n20 pp40–44
'Ongoing consent to care for older people in care homes'

Care Standards Act (2000)
HMSO

Care Standards 2003
Department of Health 2003
National minimum standards for care homes for older people. England

Chang BL (1979)
International Journal of Nursing Studies v26 pp169–182
'Locus of control, situational control and morale of the elderly'

Clough R (1981)
Old Age Homes
National Institute of Social Services Library number 44

Cooper J (2003)
Nursing and Residential Care April v5 n4 pp188–185
'Explaining the regulation of care homes in Scotland'

Copp LA (1981)
Care of the Aging
Churchill Livingstone, Edinburgh p4 Abdellah

Counsel and Care (1991)
Not Such Private Places

Counsel and Care (1992)
What if they hurt themselves?

References

Crowther MA (1981)
The Workhouse system
Methuen, London

De La Cuesta (1983)
Journal of Advanced Nursing (8) pp365–371
'The nursing process from development to implementation'

Department of Health (1998)
Our healthier nation: a contract for health

Department of Health (2001)
Essence of Care

Department of Health (2004)
Regulation of healthcare staff in England and Wales: A consultation document

Department of Health (2005)
Standard two; patient centred care

DHSS (1991)
Assessment systems and community care
HMSO

Dimon C (1995)
Elderly Care October v17 n5 p53
Preparing care assistants for the qualified invasion

Dimon C (1999a)
Nursing and Residential Care Oct v1 n7 pp412–413
Nurse knows best

Dimon C (1999b)
Equinox Issue 3 pp14–15
'Why is sexuality still a taboo subject in today's nursing homes?'

Dimon C (2002)
Nursing Standard Aug 28 v16 n50 p25
'Residents need their own charter'

Dimond B (2002)
Legal Aspects of Nursing
Prentice Hall, Hemel Hempstead

Dimond B (2005)
Nursing Times June 14 v101 n24 p18
Dilemma

Dinsdale P, Parish C (2005)

Nursing Standard April 13 v19 n31 pp15–17
'The business of caring'
Douglass RM (1992)
The Effective Nurse Leader and Manager
Mosby, USA'
Downie RS, Calman KC (1987)
Healthy Respect: Ethics in Healthcare
Faber and Faber, Oxford
Dubree M, Vogehlpohl R (1980)
American Journal of Nursing v80 n11 p2046
'When hope dies – so might the patient'
Duffin C (2000)
Nursing Standard Aug 2 v14 n46 p9
'Study finds hiding drugs in food is common practice'
English Community Care Association (2004)
Improving lives, improving life
Fiesta J (1988)
The Law and Liability: A guide for Nurses 2nd ed
J Wiley and Sons, New York
Finlay L (2005)
Nursing Management April v12 n1 pp31–35
'Difficult encounters'
Freeman MDA, Lyon CM (1984)
The Law of Residential Homes and Day Care Establishments
Sweet and Maxwell
Fry A (1992)
Nursing Times August 26 v88 n35 p 18
'A Tip of the Iceberg'
General Social Care Workforce 2002
'Codes of practice for social care workers and employers'
London
Goffman E (1961)
Asylums
Penguin, USA
Goodinson SM, Singleton J (1984)
International Journal of Nursing Studies v26 n4 pp327–341

References

'Quality of Life: A Critical Review of Current Concepts, Measures and Their Clinical Implications'
Includes Young and Longman
Goodwin S (1993)
Journal of Dementia Care 18–19 Nov/Dec
'Beyond the great care divide'
Griffiths A, Grimes RH, Roberts G (1990)
The Law and Elderly People
Routledge
Haas F (2005)
Nursing Times 18 Jan v101 n3 pp34–37
'Understanding the legal implications of living wills'
Harrison S (2004)
Nursing Standard July14 v18 n44
'Older people's specialists needed in all care homes'
Health and Safety Act (1974)
HMSO
Health and Safety Executive (1993)
Health and Safety in Residential Care Homes
HMSO (1988)
A Positive Choice
HMSO (1991)
The Children's Act 1989 Guidance and Regulations v4 Residential Care
HMSO (1992)
Confronting elder abuse
Home Office Fire Department (1983)
Draft guide to fire precautions in existing residential care premises ISBN 086 2520843
Hope KW (2004)
Dementia v3 n1 pp46–68
'Using multi-sensory environments with people with dementia'.
Human Rights Act (1998)
HMSO
James A (2004)
Nursing Times 14 Dec v100 part 50 pp228–29
'The legal and clinical implications of crushing tablet medication'

Johnson M, Hoyes L (2005)
Registering long-term care; proposals for a single registered care home
Joseph Rowntree Foundation

Kayser-Jones J, Chan J, Kris A (2005)
Geriatric Nursing v26 n1 pp16–20
'A model long-term care hospice unit: Care, Community and Compassion'

Kirkevoid O, Engedal K (2005)
Concealment of drugs in food and beverages in nursing homes: Cross sectional study
BMJ v330 January pp21–23

Laing and Buisson (1994)
Laing's Review of Private Healthcare
Laing and Buisson Publications Ltd UK

Laing and Buisson (2005)
www.laingbuisson.co.uk
April

Lane B (1993)
The encyclopaedia of cruel and unusual punishments
True Crime, London

Law Commission (1997)
'Who decides? Making decisions on behalf of mentally incapacitated adults'
Consultation paper December

Law Society and the BMJ (1995)
Guidelines for Doctors and Lawyers on the assessment of mental capacity

Longmate N (1974)
The Workhouse
Temple Smith, London

Making Decisions Alliance (2003)
Campaign Pack
www.makingdecisions.org.uk

Mason JK, McCall Smith RA (1994)
Law and Medical Ethics 4th ed
Butterworths, London p278

McGrew AG, Wilson MJ (1982)
Decision making: Aproaches and analysis
Manchester University Press

References

McPherson B (1988)
Social Work Today 22 Sept pp12–14
In Whose Best Interests?

MDA DB (2001) (04) July (2001)
Advice on the safe use of bedrails
Medicine and Healthcare Products Regulatory Agency

Meacher M (1972)
Taken For A Ride
Longman, London

Means R, Smith R (1983)
The Development of Welfare Services For Elderly People
Croom Helm, London

Menzies IEP (1970)
The functioning of social systems as a defence against anxiety
London

National Assistance Act (1948)
HMSO

National minimum standards for care homes for older people (March 2003)
Department of Health

Nazarko L (1995)
Nursing in Nursing Homes
Blackwell, Oxford

Nazarko L (1999)
Nursing Times June-July v1 n2 p24
Service Breakdown

Newton E (1979)
This Bed My Centre
Virago, London

NHS and Community Care Act (1990)
HMSO

NMC (2004)
Code of Professional Conduct
London

Norman JA (1980)
Rights and Risks
National Corporation for the Care of Older People, London

Nursing Times (1994) Jan 19 v90 n3 p8
Old People Distressed By No Pets Rule
Nursing Times (2004) Nov 2 v100 n44
Off The Record
O'Dowd A (2003)
Nursing Times 29 July v99 n30 pp10–11
Will new rules help overseas nurses?
Preston KW (1988)
Care Science and Practice v6 n4 pp116–129
'Positioning for comfort and pressure relief: The 30 degree tilt alternative'
Ramprogus V, Gibson J (1991)
Nursing Times June 20 v87 n26 pp45–47
Assessing restraint
RCN 2002
RCN Code of Practice for patient handling
RCN (2003)
Manual handling assessments in hospital and the community
Reece I, Walker S (2000)
Teaching, training and learning
Business Education Publishers Ltd, Tyne and Wear
Reed J, Stanley D (2003)
Health and Social Care in the Community v11 n4 p356–363
'Improving communication between hospitals and care homes: the development of a daily living plan for older people'
Rose ME (1971)
The English Poor Law 1780–1930
David and Charles, London
Royal Pharmaceutical Society of GB (2003)
The administration and control of medicines in care homes and children's services
Salvage J (1989)
Nursing Standard Aug 26 v48 n3
Building Centres of Excellence
Schmidt Kayser-Jones J (1981)
Old Alone and Neglected: Care of the Aged in Scotland and the USA p106

University of California Press, USA
Shea H (1986)
International Journal of Nursing Studies v23 n2
pp147–157
A Conceptual Framework to Study the Use of Nursing Care
Plans
Shields MA (2004)
The Economic Journal v114 n49 p464
'Addressing nursing shortages: What can policy makers
learn from the econometric evidence on nurse labour
supply?'
Shukla RB (ed)(1999)
Care of the elderly
Stationery Office
Skills for Care (2005)
The state of the socialcare workforce 2004
Smith BA (1977)
A History of the Nursing Profession
Heinemann
Thompson D (1983)
Ageing and Society v3 n2 pp47–69
'Workhouse to Nursing Home: Residential Care of Elderly
People in England since 1840'
Tobin SS, Lieberman MA (1976)
Last Home For The Aged
Jossey Bass USA
Townsend P (1964)
The Last Refuge
Routledge and Kegan Paul, London
UKCC (1994)
*Professional Conduct – Occasional report on standards of
nursing in nursing homes*
UKCC (2001)
Register autumn n37 p7
UKCC London (Now NMC)
Vladeck BC (1980)
Unloving Care: The Nursing Home Tragedy
USA Basic Books

Wade B, Saywer L, Bell J (1983)
Dependency with Dignity
Bedford Square Press, London
Walster D (1982)
Geriatric Medicine April pp13–19
'*Why Not Prescribe A Pet?*'
Waterlow J (1988)
Nursing Times v1 n25 pp69–70
'Prevention is cheaper than care'
Watson J (2002)
Something for everyone
British Institute of Human Rights
Weiner CL, Kayser-Jones J (1989)
Social Science and Medicine v28 n1 pp37–44
'Defensive Work in Nursing Homes: Accountability Gone Amok'
Willcocks D, Peace S, Kellaher L (1987)
Private Lives in Public Places
Tavistock, London
Wilson S (2003)
Nursing and Residential Care v5 n5 pp230–232
'The reasoning behind a good night's sleep'
Young AP (1992)
Case studies in law and nursing: A course book for project 2000 training
Chapman and Hall

BIBLIOGRAPHY

Mill JS (1974)
  On liberty
  Penguin
Nazarko L (1997)
  Nursing Times 12 Nov v93 n46 pp40–42
  A Question of Inspection
Ramprogus V, Gibson J (1991)
  Nursing Times June 20 v87 n26 pp45–47
  Assessing Restraint
Seedhouse D (1988)
  Ethics in the heart of health care
  J Wiley and Sons

APPENDIX 1

A LIST OF USEFUL ADDRESSES

AGE CONCERN, Astral House, 1268 London Road, London, SW16 4EK

ACTION ON ELDER ABUSE HELPLINE. 0808 808 8141

BRITISH INSTITUTE OF HUMAN RIGHTS, Law School, King's College London, 26-29 Drury Lane, London, WC1B 5RL. 02078481818

COMMISSION FOR SOCIAL CARE INSPECTION, 33 Greycoat Street, London, SW1P 2Q. 0845 0150120

COUNSEL AND CARE, Twyman House, 16 Bonny Street, London, NW1 9PG. 0207241 8555

GENERAL SOCIAL CARE COUNCIL, Golding's House, 2 Hay's Lane, London, SE1 2HB. 0207397 5100

HEALTH AND SAFETY EXECUTIVE, Information Centre, Broad Lane, Sheffield, 53 7HG

HELP THE AGED, 207-221 Pentonville Road, London. 0207 2781114

HUMAN RIGHTS UNIT HELPDESK, Home Office, 50 Queen Anne's Gate, London, SW1H 9AT

MAKING DECISIONS ALLIANCE, c/o Turning Point, Newloom House, 101 Black Church Lane, London, EC1 1LU

NMC (Nursing Midwifery Council), 23 Portland Place, London, W13 1P2. Advice line: 0207 333 6760

PUBLIC GUARDIAN OFFICE. 0207 664 7000

RCN, 20 Cavendish Square, London, W1G ORN. 020 7409 3333

Advice is available from special interest forums such as INFORM or the Care of Older People.

ROSEMONT PHARMACEUTICALS. *For advice on liquid medication.* 0800 919312

Bibliography

ROYAL PHARMACEUTICAL SOCIETY OF GREAT
BRITAIN, 1 Lambeth High Street, London, SE1 7JN.
0207 572 2409

APPENDIX 2

CARE PLAN AUDIT

1 Is black ink used?   YES ☐   NO ☐

2 Are the entries   a) signed?   YES ☐   NO ☐

                      b) dated?   YES ☐   NO ☐

                      c) timed?   YES ☐   NO ☐

3 Is the assessment form
   completed within 1 week of
   admission?   YES ☐   NO ☐

4 Is the care plan completed within
   7 days of admission?   YES ☐   NO ☐

5 Are all the forms completed   YES ☐   NO ☐

   a) waterlow   YES ☐   NO ☐

   b) nutrition   YES ☐   NO ☐

   c) manual handling   YES ☐   NO ☐

   d) bedside risk assessment   YES ☐   NO ☐

   e) fall risk assessment   YES ☐   NO ☐

   f) profile assessment   YES ☐   NO ☐

Appendices

g) others   YES ☐   NO ☐

6 Are all problems identified?   YES ☐   NO ☐

7 Have residents/relatives signed the
   care plan?   YES ☐   NO ☐

8 Is the care plan evaluated monthly? YES ☐   NO ☐

9 Are problems and risk assessments
   re-written yearly?   YES ☐   NO ☐

10 Are progress notes written in?   YES ☐   NO ☐

11 Do care assistants make additions
   to care plans?   YES ☐   NO ☐

12 Is the key worker diary written in?   YES ☐   NO ☐

13 Are visit forms completed?   YES ☐   NO ☐

APPENDIX 3

RISK ASSESSMENT

NAME:

DATE OF BIRTH:

Need or wish of resident:

State risks involved;

To resident:

To others:

To the nurse or care assistant:

What will be done to reduce the risks:

Re-assessment and evaluation:

Printed in the United Kingdom
by Lightning Source UK Ltd.
124695UK00001B/79-141/A